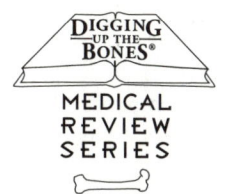

MEDICAL
REVIEW
SERIES

Pathology

Notice

Medicine is an ever-changing science. As new research and clinical experience broaden our knowledge, changes in treatment and drug therapy are required. The author and the publisher of this work have checked with sources believed to be reliable in their efforts to provide information that is complete and generally in accord with the standards accepted at the time of publication. However, in view of the possibility of human error or changes in medical sciences, neither the author, nor the publisher, nor any other party who has been involved in the preparation or publication of this work warrants that the information contained herein is in every respect accurate or complete and they are not responsible for any errors or omissions or for the results obtained from use of such information. Readers are encouraged to confirm the information contained herein with other sources. For example and in particular, readers are advised to check the product information sheet included in the package of each drug they plan to administer to be certain that the information contained in this book is accurate and that changes have not been made in the recommended dose or in the contraindications for administration. This recommendation is of particular importance in connection with new or infrequently used drugs.

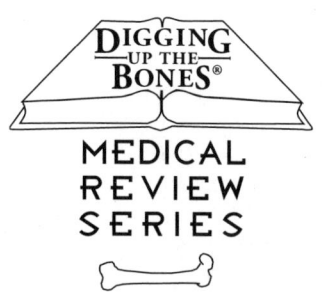

Pathology

Second Edition

Compiled and Written by
Nikos M. Linardakis, M.D.

McGraw-Hill
Health Professions Division

New York St. Louis San Francisco Auckland Bogotá Caracas Lisbon
London Madrid Mexico City Milan Montreal New Delhi San Juan
Singapore Sydney Tokyo Toronto

McGraw-Hill
A Division of The **McGraw·Hill** Companies

PATHOLOGY: Digging Up the Bones

Copyright ©1998 by *The **McGraw-Hill** Companies, Inc.* All rights reserved. Printed in the United States of America. Except as permitted under the United States Copyright Act of 1976, no part of this publication may be reproduced or distributed in any form or by any means, or stored in a date base or retrieval system, without prior written permission of the publisher.

1234567890 MAL MAL 9987

ISBN 0-07-038216-6

This book was set in Times Roman by V & M Graphics, Inc.
The editors were John Dolan and Steven Melvin;
the production supervisor was Helene G. Landers;
the cover designer was Mathew Dvorozniak.

Malloy Lithographing, Inc., was the printer and binder.

Cataloging-in-Publication Data is on file for this title at the Library of Congress

To my brothers, John, Dino, and Christos

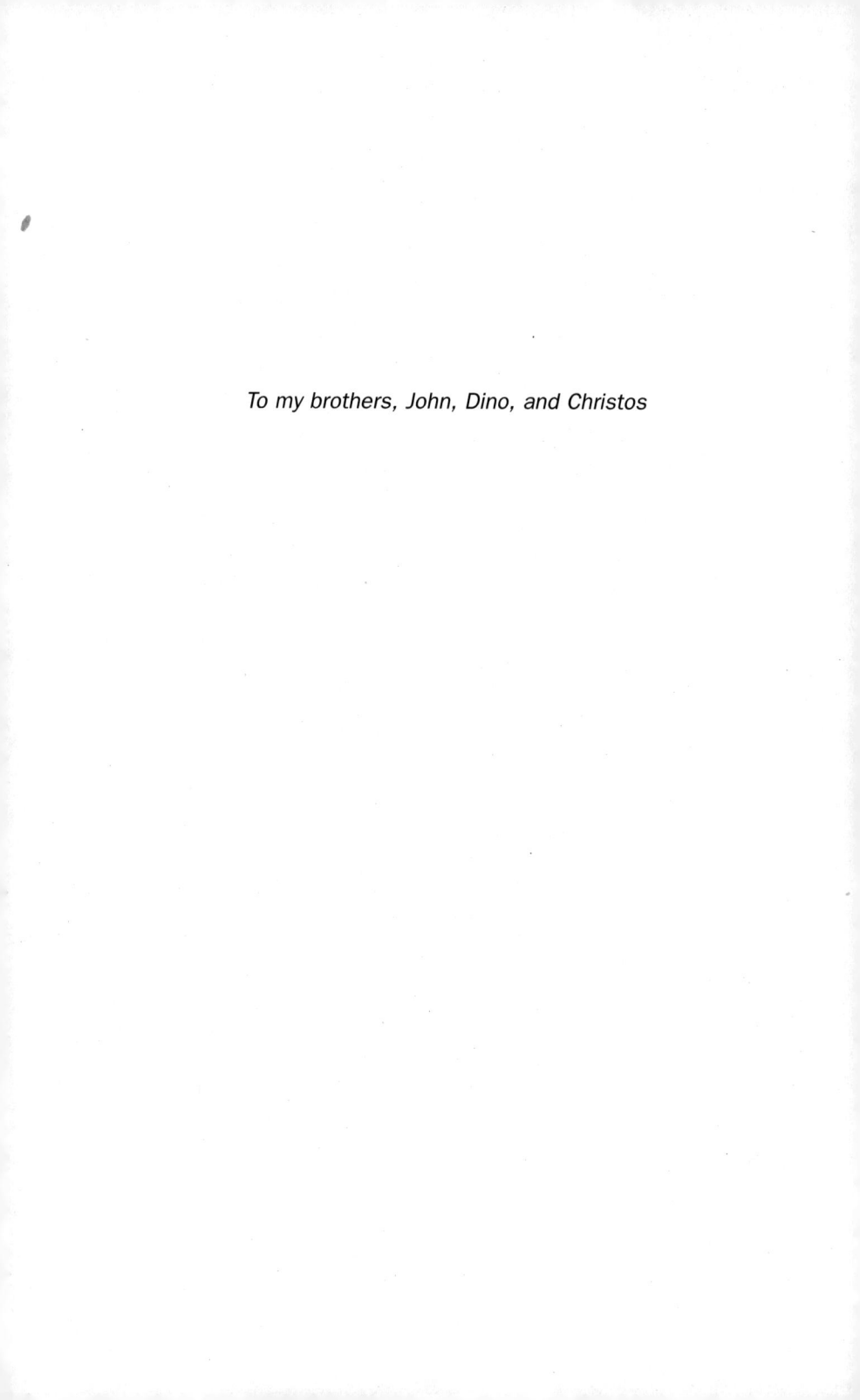

Contents

Preface   ix

Chapter 1
General Pathology — 1

Chapter 2
Hematology/Cells — 7

Chapter 3
Cardiovascular — 27

Chapter 4
Gastrointestinal — 35

Chapter 5
Respiratory — 49

Chapter 6
Endocrine — 59

Chapter 7
Nervous System — 67

Chapter 8
Genitourinary 73

Chapter 9
Skin/Breast 85

Chapter 10
Musculoskeletal 91

Chapter 11
Syndromes 97

Chapter 12
Miscellaneous 105

Index 117

Note 127

Color Plates

Preface

Many people have asked how the *Digging Up the Bones* medical review series was created. Because I want everyone to benefit from the books, let me take a moment to discuss the development of the series. We wanted to find every exam, every question, every opportunity that would lead in the direction of understanding *where* to begin, *what* questions were going to be asked, *which* topics were repeatedly covered, *why* certain facts were important to highlight on an exam, and *when* to say "I've studied that, and I know the answer!"

This review series evolved with the time, knowledge, and interviews with doctors, clinicians, professors, and finding the *bare bones essentials* to the medical school curriculum. In collaboration with several students, authors, professors, and editors, we *dig up the bones* of the different areas for the past 9 years to bring these concepts in front of you—in a quick, focused approach. Thus, the purpose of this series is to restate, illustrate, and focus on the *significant* material for your coursework, exams, and future working career in medicine.

After its creation, a few other "high-yield quick" review books have been generated, but they do not put the same emphasis on the review presented to you as in the *Digging Up the Bones* medical review series. With each title, you should feel confident that you have covered the highest-tested areas—which are most likely to appear on your exams.

Absorb as much as you can. Carry that deep desire to learn everything in these books, review them repeatedly (reread each book at least twice; you'll be amazed at how much things make more sense after going through it a couple of times), learn to *recognize* items as well as memorizing them, think things through, share the book with a colleague and talk about things to help in the memory game. And remember, make your learning as active a process as you can.

I want your comments, feedback, additional items to include in the future. You are acquiring an incredible amount of material in medicine, now we will focus on the highly tested areas. This series is addictive, and every part of learning should be this way. When you really love something, you get involved. Now that you have the information, good luck with everything. I know you will feel more confident about the topics, and will be prepared for your exams.

So, let us begin!

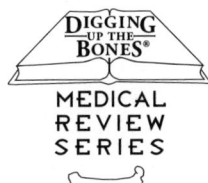

Pathology

General Pathology

1

In this second edition of *Pathology*, we have added several illustrations and tables to highlight areas typically covered on board and course examinations. Furthermore, the additions made include material covered on past examinations. When you take a future exam, pay attention to the *clinical scenario* when answering a question with a slide or gross photo. You will notice that several of the questions can be answered *prior to* even looking at the photo—just by reading the clinical presentation. On the other hand, paying attention to specific areas in a slide or photo may answer the question without a doubt. Remember, "a picture is worth a thousand words." Please take the time to study the included illustrations, these are *important* review items. In *pathology*, we study medicine in its relation to disease and abnormal conditions. We emphasize topics in this book to offer a summary of the highly tested words, associations, concepts, and laboratory findings in pathology. Now, let's begin.

"MALIGNANCY" = Metastasis and invasion.

Malignant cells have increased locomotive properties, and decreased cohesiveness. Malignant cell transformation includes: loss of contact-inhibition of growth, "immortality," increased transplantability, and a *decreased* dependency on exogenous growth factors. Metastasis is the development of cancer (implants) into distant tissues. Remember, carcinogenic promoters *alone* are NOT carcinogenic. Instead, tumor promoters "promote" cell proliferation (they do NOT *directly* induce DNA damage).

MALIGNANT TRANSFORMATIONS
Point mutation—**ras** gene in carcinoma of *colon*.
Chromosomal translocation—**c-myc** and immunoglobulin *heavy* chain genes in *Burkitt's Lymphoma*.
Gene amplification—**N-myc** gene in *Neuroblastoma*.
Gene deletion or inactivation—**rb** gene in **R**etinoblastoma.

PRECANCEROUS LESIONS: solar keratosis of skin, leukoplakia of oral cavity, familial multiple polyposis, and chronic atrophic gastritis of pernicious anemia. These also have malignant potential: adenomatous polyps, *villous* adenomas, and colonic dysplasia (NOT hyperplastic polyp, nor Peutz-Jeghers syndrome).

MALIGNANT NEOPLASMS INCLUDE: seminoma, melanoma, myelocytic leukemia, papillary carcinoma of the thyroid gland, osteogenic sarcoma, and squamous cell carcinoma of the skin.

SYSTEMIC MANIFESTATIONS OF NEOPLASMS
These include: migratory thrombophlebitis, fever, pruritus, galactorrhea.

CANCERS metastasize via *Lymphatics*.

SARCOMAS metastasize via *Hematogenous spread* (through blood). Sarcomas are malignant neoplasms from tissues of *mesenchymal origin*.

MALIGNANT FIBROUS HISTIOCYTOMAS
Common in elderly. These are about one quarter of all sarcomas. They are most common in the extremities, and have immune markers, α-1-antitrypsin, and factor 8 antigen.

CHALONES
Hypothetical substances that physiologically restrain cell proliferation (it is a tissue-specific mitotic inhibitor). They are found in normal tissue, and inhibit hyperplasia.

NERVE GROWTH FACTOR
This growth factor may stimulate wound healing.

ECCHYMOSES
This is another term for common *bruises*.

DEFICIENCY OF FAT-SOLUBLE VITAMINS
Total obstruction of the common bile duct, and severe pancreatic insufficiency will result in an impaired absorption of the fat-soluble vitamins (A, D, E, and K).

VITAMIN A
Vitamin A plays important roles in reproduction, growth, and epithelial tissue upkeep. Deficiency results in impaired night vision, "night blindness," as well as xerophthalmia. Vitamin A deficiency may lead to the

development of complicated infections in the respiratory tract, eyes, and urinary tract (NOT the central nervous system). Deficiency may cause the male to be unable to form sperm cells, and may retard growth. Vitamin A maintains epithelial tissues and avoids corneal atrophy.

β-carotene can form 2 retinal molecules, it may also decrease the risk for lung cancer and other carcinomas.

VITAMIN D

Vitamin D is the most toxic vitamin. A *deficiency* of Vitamin D in children is called Rickets. A deficiency in adults is called Osteomalacia.

VITAMIN E

(*Least* toxic fat-soluble vitamin.) High doses of Vitamin E may decrease the risk for coronary artery disease.

VITAMIN K

Vitamin K acts as a cofactor for prothrombin and clotting factors 7, 9, and 10 in blood coagulation. Toxicity may cause hemolytic anemia and jaundice. A deficiency may cause a decreased carboxylation of the glutamic acid residues of prothrombin, and a decreased formation of fibrin monomers (from fibrinogen). Also, a deficiency may cause a decrease in the binding of Ca^{++} to prothrombin (factor II). Bacteria in the intestine make Vitamin K except in newborns or when undergoing antimicrobial therapy, this is a reason newborns receive a shot of Vitamin K.

DEFICIENCY OF WATER-SOLUBLE VITAMINS

These are the remaining vitamins which include: B vitamins, biotin, pantothenic acid, folic acid, and ascorbic acid.

VITAMIN B$_1$ (THIAMINE)

Deficiency can result in *Beri-beri* and Wernicke-Korsakoff Syndrome.

VITAMIN B$_2$ (RIBOFLAVIN)

Deficiency results in dermatitis, glossitis, and cheilosis (cracking at the corner of the mouth).

VITAMIN B$_6$ (PYRIDOXINE)

Deficiency is associated with Isoniazid anti-tuberculosis treatment (therefore, pyridoxine is given). In general, *water*-soluble vitamins are not usually toxic, but this is actually a toxic vitamin that can result in gait problems from CNS toxicity.

VITAMIN B$_{12}$ (COBALAMIN)

Vitamin B$_{12}$ binds to intrinsic factor for absorption. A deficiency results from decreased parietal cell secretion of intrinsic factor (IF) in the stomach, causing *pernicious megaloblastic anemia*. This is due to decreased

IF, and therefore decreased absorption of vitamin B_{12}. Vitamin B_{12} deficiency will also cause *neurologic problems* (folate deficiency only results in megaloblastic anemia).

NIACIN (NICOTINIC ACID)
A deficiency results in *Pellagra*: **d**ermatitis, **d**iarrhea, and **d**ementia (the "3-D's"). The skin lesion is the earliest sign of pellagra—for example, phototoxic dermatitis.

BIOTIN
The only deficiency may appear with eating a diet of raw egg whites (that have avidin). *Avidin* prevents absorption by binding to biotin.

FOLIC ACID
Deficiency results in *megaloblastic anemia* (frequently seen in alcoholics and pregnant women; very common). Pregnant women must receive folic acid *early* in fetal development to avoid *neural tube defects* (i.e., spina bifida) and growth failure. It is recommended to begin vitamin supplements *before* conception.

Folate deficiency is associated with: oval macrocytosis, hypersegmented polyps, megaloblastic erythropoiesis, leukopenia, and thrombocytopenia (NOT subacute combined degeneration nor posterolateral degeneration—these are neurologic changes associated with vitamin B_{12} deficiency).

ASCORBIC ACID (VITAMIN C)
Excretion of increased levels of vitamin C may result in kidney stones by calcium salt deposits of oxalate (a breakdown product). Deficiency results in *scurvy*: deficient hydroxylation of collagen and therefore, connective tissue problems which include sore gums and loose teeth, as well as anemia. Ascorbic acid deficiency may delay the healing of abscesses. Vitamin C deficiency impairs the synthesis of type II collagen (cartilage)—NOT type I (bone) collagen.

Deficiency	Causes
Vitamin A	Xerophthalmia, Night Blindness
Vitamin D	Rickets in children, Osteomalacia in adults. Causes an excess of osteoid tissue.
Vitamin E	(Usually in *premature* infants)

Deficiency	Causes
Vitamin K	(Deficiency is unusual for an adult), Hemorrhagic disease of the newborn, Decreased prothrombin level, Prolonged coagulation time.
Fat-Soluble Vitamins (A, D, E, and K)	Steatorrhea of Cystic Fibrosis
Vitamin B_1 (Thiamine)	Beri-beri (from polished rice as diet) characterized by dry skin and irritability, with eventual death. (therefore, must treat) Wernicke-Korsakoff Syndrome (seen in chronic alcoholics) Affects the Peripheral and Central Nervous Systems. Affects the circulatory system. (NO effect on the digestive system)
Vitamin B_2 (Riboflavin)	Dermatitis, Glossitis, and Cheilosis
Vitamin B_6 (Pyridoxine)	(Associated with Isoniazid anti-tuberculosis treatment) **Micro**cytic anemia
Vitamin B_{12} (Cobalamin)	Pernicious megaloblastic anemia (From lack of intrinsic factor), Neurologic problems.
Niacin (Nicotinic acid)	Pellagra: "3 D's" **D**ermatitis, **D**iarrhea, and **D**ementia Neuropsychiatric syndrome.
Biotin	Lethargy, acidosis, and dehydration; Increased urine levels of propionic acid, and increased intermediates of isoleucine intermediates. Caused from a diet of raw egg whites (that have avidin)

(continued)

(Continued)

Deficiency	Causes
Folate	Megaloblastic anemia (**Macro**cytic anemia), Neural tube defects in children of deficient pregnant mother. Increased formiminoglutamic acid in urine after patient is given Histidine.
Ascorbic acid (Vitamin C)	Scurvy (Connective tissue problems; sore gums and loose teeth) Perifollicular petechiae, Difficult wound healing by decreased hydroxylation of lysine and proline.

Hematology/Cells 2

INFLAMMATION

Caused by: bacteria, cell necrosis, viruses, and thermal injury. In *acute* inflammation, look for large numbers of PMNs, serous exudate, fibrinous exudate, purulent exudate, vasodilation (but, NO granuloma formation). Hageman factor, prostaglandins, bradykinin, and fibrolysin play a role in the *initiation, development and resolution* of an acute inflammatory response. There is usually: an increase in oncotic pressure of interstitial fluid, vasodilation and widened interendothelial gaps, and decreased blood flow. Potent *chemotactic agents* or mediators: **C5a** and **Leukotriene B$_4$** (NOT C3a and PGE$_2$).

It is elicited by liquefaction and coagulation necrosis, trauma, or microbes. Slowing of blood flow with margination of cells, migration of neutrophils through vessel walls, enzymatic digestion of necrotic debris (but, NOT dissolution of vascular basement membrane).

CHRONIC INFLAMMATORY CELLS (Fig. 2-1)

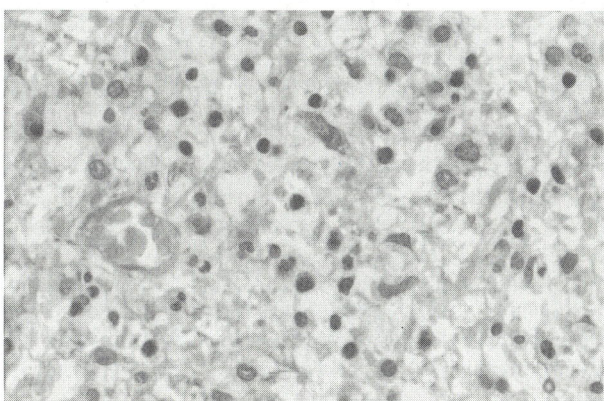

Figure 2-1 Inflammatory cells (macrophages, plasma cells, and lymphocytes) respond to tissue damage, inflammation, and persistent damaging factors. Chronic inflammation can lead to scarring. (For color version see Color Plate 1.)

White Blood Cells
Neutrophils > Lymphocytes > Monocytes > Eosinophils > Basophils

Neutrophils
These cells are also known as polymorphonucleocytes (PMNs). They are the main white blood cells of *acute* inflammation. They arrive at the site of injury by chemotaxis and act by phagocytosis and then release the lysosomal enzymes (myeloperoxidase, acid hydrolases, lysozyme, and proteases).

PMNs occur with: acute inflammation, lobar pneumonia, malignancy, and myocardial infarction (NOT whooping cough).

Bactericidal activity includes: Increased pentose phosphate pathway, production of superoxide radicals, halogenation of bacteria, and production of H_2O_2. They are mobile and more numerous in circulating blood (and are NOT long-lived, and NOT resistant to decreased pH).

Basophils
These cells are *basophilic* and thus, stain blue. They participate in type I hypersensitivity reactions by stimulating the production of Ig**E**, and then release *histamine* and SRS-A (slow-reacting substance of anaphylaxis). An increase in basophils in the peripheral blood smear is associated with: Polycythemia vera, Chronic myeloid *leukemia* (CML), and myeloid metaplasia.

Eosinophils
These *bilobed* nucleated cells are *eosinophilic* and thus, stain reddish. They contain hydrolytic enzymes. They increase in parasitic infections.

Macrophages
These include macrophages, Kupffer cells (in the liver), histiocytes (in connective tissue), and mesangial cells (in the kidney). *Monocytes* develop into macrophages. They act by phagocytosis (engulf particles), and pinocytosis (engulf fluid with the particles). The lysosomal digestion will degrade and act against microorganisms.

Lymphocytes
These cells increase following the PMNs and are considered T cells and B cells. T cells developed from the *thymus*, and B cells developed from the *bursa of Fabricus* (in birds). B cells differentiate into *plasma cells* which produce immunoglobulins (e.g., IgG).

Null Cells
These include lymphocytes like Natural Killer (NK) cells and Killer (K) cells. These cells act in transplant rejection and in the defense mechanism for viral infections.

CHEMICAL MEDIATORS

HISTAMINE
Mast cells contain the majority of histamine (basophils and platelets also contain histamine). Histamine is released by mast cell degranulation. Histamine release is stimulated by: physical injury, like trauma or heat; antibody-mediated immunologic reactions; C3a and C5a complement products; and neutrophilic lysosomal proteins. The degranulation will allow histamine to have an *initial* vasoconstriction, then vaso**dilation**.

BRADYKININ
Both bradykinin and histamine will increase vascular permeability. Bradykinin causes an increase in vascular permeability, vasoconstriction, and *pain*. Bradykinin causes arteriolar dilation and endothelial contraction with widening of venular interendothelial gaps. It also increases phospholipases and arachidonic acid release.

PHAGOCYTIC CELLS
Phagocytic cells include: monocytes, mesangial cells, microglia, and macrophages like Kupffer cells (NOT plasma cells).

NUMBER OF T-CELLS > NUMBER OF B-CELLS IN:
Paracortical areas of lymph nodes, peripheral blood, and periarteriolar sheaths of spleen. (As a rule, B-cells are the *follicular* centers of lymph *nodes*.)

GIANT CELL
This is formed as a fusion of *histiocytes*. Inflammatory giant cells are derived from the cytoplasmic fusion of epithelioid cells (NOT foreign body giant cells).

INFLAMMATORY EDEMA
In inflammatory edema, we can see: *increased* blood flow in regional lymphatics, increased interstitial fluid oncotic pressure, and *decreased* intravascular oncotic pressure. Edema may result from: *increased* capillary hydrostatic pressure, increased capillary permeability, increased cardiac output, protein calorie malnutrition, and *decreased* plasma oncotic pressure.

ASCITES
This is considered the pathologic presence of fluid in the peritoneal cavity.

VITAMIN K

This vitamin is a cofactor to *increase* formation of factors II, VII, IX, and X.

FACTOR VII (7)

This factor is active in the *extrinsic* blood coagulation cascade.

FACTOR VIIIC (8C) DEFICIENCY

This is also known as Classic hemophilia or Hemophilia **A**. It is an X-linked disorder and is associated with von Willebrand's disease, disseminated intravascular coagulations (DIC). It is probably caused by a combined primary (failure of platelet *adhesion*), and a secondary (*lack of factor* 8c) hemostatic defect. It is associated with bleeding into muscles, subcutaneous tissue, and joints. Look for a prolonged activated partial thromboplastin time in Classic hemophilia.

FACTOR IX (9) DEFICIENCY

This is also known as Hemophilia **B** or Christmas Disease. It is an X-linked disorder and is associated with prolonged activated partial thromboplastin time (APTT). (But, NOT prolonged bleeding time, NOR prolonged thrombin time.)

HAGEMAN FACTOR (FACTOR 12)

This factor is active in both the intrinsic blood coagulation enzyme cascade and the kallikrein system.

PLATELET RELEASE REACTION (Fig. 2-2)

Calcium, Serotonin, ADP, and Thromboglobulin are released.

BLEEDING TIME

This is the measured time to assess *platelet function*, adhesion, and vascular factors in blood clotting.

PROTHROMBIN TIME (PT)

The prothrombin time allows us to screen for abnormalities of factors II (prothrombin), V, **VII**, X, and fibrinogen. It is a widely used measure of the **extrinsic** pathway of coagulation. Add an excess of calcium and tissue factor to test the plasma, and measure the time to form a clot.

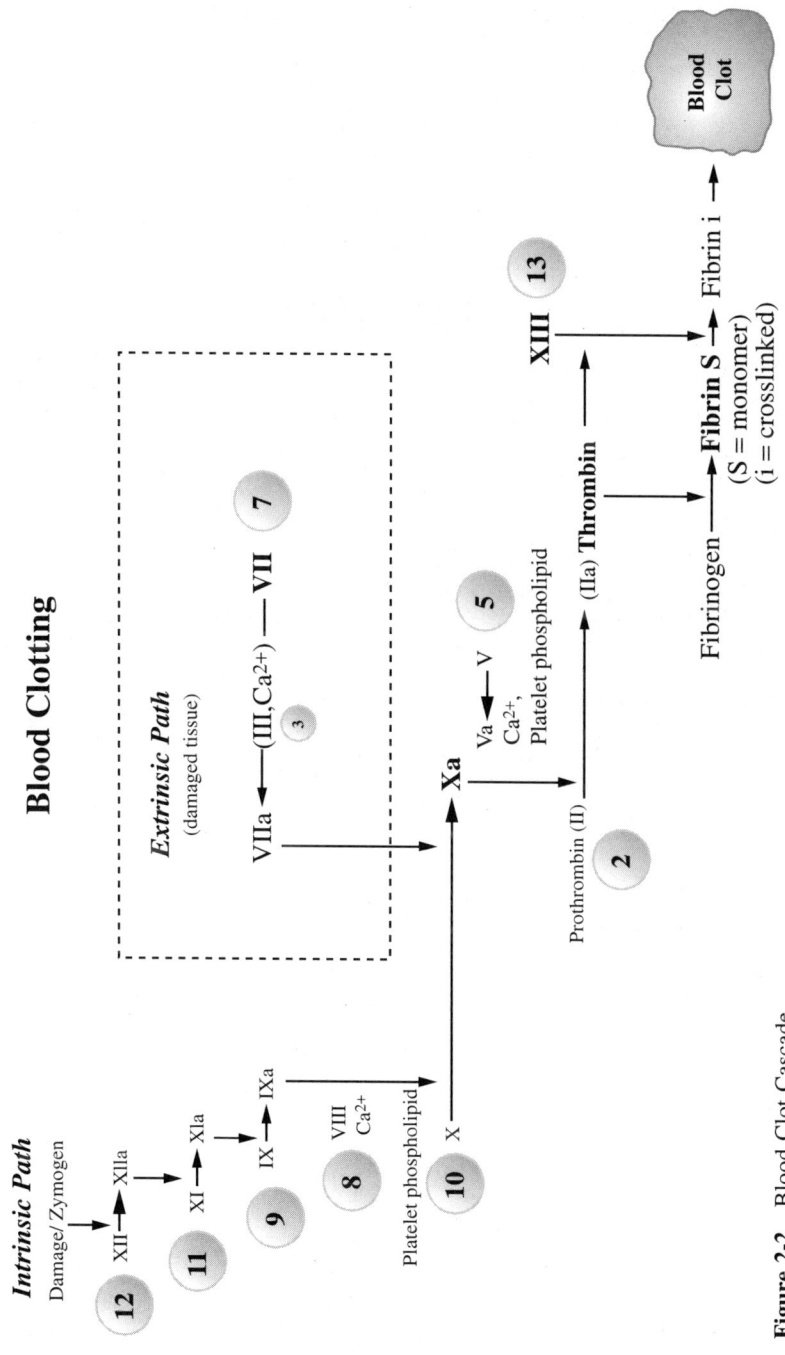

Figure 2-2 Blood Clot Cascade.

ACTIVATED PARTIAL THROMBOPLASTIN TIME (APTT)

APTT allows the screening of blood factors. It will detect abnormalities of the **in**trinsic factors: **VIIIc**, IX, X, XI, and XII (NOT VII, and XIII). APTT is *prolonged* with: Classic hemophilia, von Willebrand's disease, or Christmas disease (but, NOT with long-term treatment with aspirin).

The Intrinsic Pathway requires factors V, VIII, X, and XII. It does NOT require factor VII—like the extrinsic Pathway.

THROMBOCYTOPENIA

Thrombocytopenia is a decrease in platelets causing petechial bleeding, and it occurs with: acute leukemia, aplastic anemia, DIC (disseminated intravascular coagulation), pernicious anemia (but, NOT with polycythemia vera). It is associated with: *petechiae* and drug-induced thrombocytopenia (i.e., from methotrexate).

Thrombotic thrombocytopenic purpura (TTP) is a syndrome that includes: thrombocytopenia, hemolytic anemia, with fragmented red blood cells, helmet cells, and schistocytes. Furthermore TTP is associated with: neurologic abnormalities, renal insufficiency, fever, and a prolonged bleeding time. (It does NOT have a decreased reticulocyte count.)

Idiopathic thrombocytopenic purpura (ITP) is an immunologically mediated destruction of platelets (autoantibodies) that occurs in the spleen. ITP is associated with other autoimmune disorders (i.e., SLE), and appears with petechial hemorrhages.

VON WILLEBRAND'S DISEASE

This occurs through autosomal dominant inheritance as deficiency of von Willebrand's Factor (vWF). It presents as *decreased* factor VIIIc activity (procoagulant VIIIc). There is a *prolonged* bleeding time and activated partial thromboplastin time (APTT)—(but, NOT a prolonged PT).

Von Willebrand's Factor is synthesized by **endo**thelial cells and megakaryocytes. It is considered a large **c**arrier protein for factor VIII. It also allows platelets to *adhere* to the subendothelium when there is injury to a vessel. Therefore, vWF is important in *platelet adhesion* (NOT for platelet contraction, aggregation, nor the release reaction).

POLYCYTHEMIA VERA

Polycythemia is an *increase* in the red cell mass by proliferation of the red cells. This is a thrombotic phenomena that progresses to a late leukemia phase in most cases. It may end acute leukemia. Signs and symptoms include: splenomegaly, cyanotic (from deoxygenation of peripheral blood—NOT oxygen desaturation), abdominal pain (splenorenal infarcts), and symptomatic gout. Polycythemia is either primary, like polycythemia vera (marrow proliferation), or secondary (increased red cell mass as a reaction to hypoxia or other cause of increased erythropoietin). It is uncommon and affects the elderly. Polycythemia vera is associated with: *myelofibrosis*, anemia, leukemia, and may lead to heart failure or MI. On lab examination, the erythropoietin level is normal, but the total erythrocyte count is elevated and there is a *high* hematocrit.

PRIMARY HEMOSTASIS DISORDERS

Deficiency of *platelet plug formation.*

SECONDARY HEMOSTASIS DISORDERS

Deficiency of plasma *clotting factors*.

PLATELET AGGREGATION

Aggregation is *excited* by: ADP, thromboxane A_2, and thrombin. It is inhibited by prostacyclin.

CYCLOOXYGENASE PATHWAY

One of the two principle pathways of prostaglandin synthesis. Produces factors that can affect platelets and leukocytes. Can be blocked by aspirin or indomethacin. This pathway is initiated by the activation of phospholipase.

ASPIRIN

Aspirin prevents coronary artery disease by inhibiting the synthesis of Thromboxane A_2 *more* than inhibiting prostacyclin synthesis. Therefore, there is more prostacyclin. Overall, aspirin decreases Thromboxane (TXA_2), Prostacyclin (PGI_2), and Prostaglandin (PGE_2) (it does NOT decrease leukotrienes—*see diagram*). Aspirin treatment is aimed at cyclooxygenase inhibition of platelet aggregation in the arterial circulation.

LIPOXYGENASE PATHWAY PRODUCTS

Arachidonic acid metabolism in the lipoxygenase pathway will produce the following: HETE, SRS-A (slow reacting substance of anaphylaxis), LTC_4, LTD_4, and LTE_4 (NOT Thromboxane A_2, nor Prostacyclin) (Fig. 2-3).

Prostaglandin & Leukotriene Synthesis

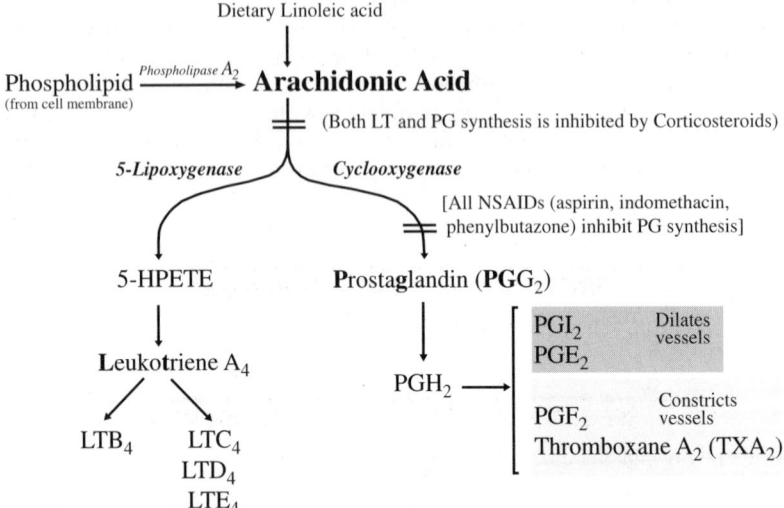

Figure 2-3 Aspirin inhibits the enzyme *Cyclooxygenase*. It therefore inhibits the synthesis of prostaglandins and thromboxanes. As you can see from the diagram, it does NOT inhibit *lipoxygenase* nor the synthesis of leukotrienes.

DISSEMINATED INTRAVASCULAR COAGULATION (DIC)

DIC occurs when there is a large, prevalent clotting that uses the platelets and coagulation factors. This overuse of clotting factors subsequently results in platelet and blood factor deficiency, and *hemorrhage* occurs. The bleeding time, PT, thrombin time, APTT are all *prolonged*.

DIC can be caused by the following clinical scenarios: *toxemia*, with bacteremia (infection) by gram-negative organisms, amniotic fluid emboli, premature separation of the placenta or abruptio placenta, cancer, trauma, and other hemolytic anemia problems (but, NOT by *peripheral* venous thrombosis).

ENDOTHELIAL THROMBORESISTANCE

Mediated by: heparan sulfate, thrombomodulin, tissue plasminogen activator (TPA), and prostacyclin (PGI_2), NOT ADP. Heparan sulfate is an endothelial proteoglycan that activates antithrombin.

IRREVERSIBLE CELL INJURY AND NECROSIS

Nuclear changes in cell death:

KARYOLYSIS
There is a fading to the chromatin substance.

PYKNOSIS
The basophilic chromatin begins to degenerate and form clumps.

KARYORRHEXIS
The chromatin becomes fragmented.

NUCLEAR DISAPPEARANCE
No nucleus is visible.

Site	Types of Necrosis
Lung	This organ may produce *red infarcts* or *hemorrhagic necrosis*.
Brain, Abscesses	This organ may undergo *liquefactive necrosis*.
Heart, Kidney, Liver	These organs may undergo *coagulation necrosis*.
Tuberculous Lesions	Caseous Necrosis

CELL INJURY AND ADAPTATION

Endocrine tissue increases mass by hyper**plasia** (NOT hyper*trophy*). Hyper**trophy** (NOT hyper*plasia*) is most commonly seen in differentiated cells that do **not** secrete macromolecules. Normal tissues may have metastatic calcification. Mallory bodies are a collection of intermediate filaments in liver cells. Serum enzymes are useful to quantify because the enzymes are released more from injured or dead cells than from normal cells.

METASTATIC CALCIFICATION

Metastatic calcification is seen in calcification of the *normal* tissues. The calcium salts are deposited in *living* tissues, and there is always an *increased* concentration of blood calcium—hypercalcemia. This may occur in hyperparathyroidism, increased vitamin D, and Addison's.

DYSTROPHIC CALCIFICATION

Calcium deposits in necrotic (dead or dying) tissue. The calcium levels are *normal*. This may occur in caseous necrosis, old scars, and in damaged heart valves (*old* disease).

METAPLASIA

This is the abnormal *transformation* of a type of tissue into a differentiated tissue (of another kind). For example, as a *change* of epithelial surface in the bronchus of a heavy smoker.

RETICULOCYTES

Reticulocytes are *young* red blood cells. There will be an increased "retic count" in peripheral blood with the following associated conditions: increased red blood cell production, polychromasia and polychromatophilia, hemolytic anemia, and hemorrhage (*normal* reticulocyte count is <1 percent of all red blood cells). Reticulocyte count is a lab test used as a clinical measure of the *red blood cell production*.

TUMOR STAGING

TNM = **T**umor, **N**ode, **M**etastases
Staging is more useful (than tumor grading) for the prognosis of a cancer. It tells the tumor *size*, lymph *node* involvement, and whether there are *metastases*.

TUMOR GRADING

Grading from I to IV will offer another tool for the prognosis of a tumor. The *higher* the grade, the *more aggressive* the tumor—and worse the prognosis. It "grades" the *degree of differentiation* (amount of anaplasia and invasion).

CANCERS OF VIRAL ETIOLOGY

Burkitt's Lymphoma (African type) is associated with Epstein-Barr Virus (EBV).
Nasopharyngeal carcinoma is associated with EBV.
Carcinoma of the cervix and vulva is associated with human papilloma virus (HPV).
Adult T-cell leukemia and lymphoma is associated with HTLV-I.
Kaposi's sarcoma is associated with human immunodeficiency virus (HIV).
Hepatocellular carcinoma is associated with hepatitis B virus (HBV).

HODGKIN'S DISEASE (HD) (Fig. 2-4)

The *stage* (NOT the grade) of the disease, at diagnosis, is more useful in determining the *prognosis* in HD. The *stage* will indicate the plans for *therapy*. The histiologic type is also important. The most aggressive and worst prognosis of HD is *lymphocytic depletion*. If we look at the types of HD, we will recognize that the best-to-worst prognoses are as follows: Lymphocytic *predominance*

→ Nodular sclerosis → Mixed cellularity → Lymphocytic *depletion*. HD usually presents as a *single group* of affected nodes; for example in the para-aortic area or cervical area, etc.

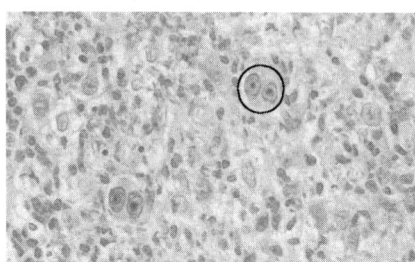

Figure 2-4 Hodgkin's disease. Reed-Sternberg cells (*circled*), which resemble owl eyes. (For color version see Color Plate 2.)

NON-HODGKIN'S LYMPHOMA

These malignant lymphomas are fairly common. They are associated with viruses, chemicals, chromosomal abnormalities, and infection. Several of the non-Hodgkin's lymphomas are associated with other diseases. The following should be memorized:

Non-Hodgkin's Lymphoma	Associated with
Well-differentiated, lymphocytic (small) lymphoma	CLL
Small lymphocyte lymphoma, plasmacytoid	Waldenstrom's Macroglobulinemia
Lymphoblastic lymphoma	T-ALL
Burkitt's Lymphoma	B-ALL t(8;14) (t = translocation)
Poorly-differentiated, lymphocytic (follicular, predominantly small cleaved-cell lymphoma)	(SLL > leukemia), t(14;18)
Adult T-Cell Leukemia/lymphoma	HTLV-1 infection

Non-Hodgkin's lymphoma usually presents with *extranodal involvement*, and *multiple groups* of affected peripheral nodes.

NODULAR, POORLY DIFFERENTIATED LYMPHOCYTIC LYMPHOMA

These are considered follicular lymphomas and include: *Follicular*, predominantly *small cleaved-cell lymphoma*. The poorly differentiated lymphomas are most frequent in the elderly. They have a characteristic paratrabecular pattern of bone marrow involvement. It occurs by a translocation at the 14 and 18 gene locations; **t(14;18)** translocation. There is an increased expression of **Bcl-2** oncogene. It presents as a slow, pain**less** course, but it is *difficult* to treat. As such, this is NOT considered an aggressive lymphoma. It is NOT a high grade classification in working formulation.

BURKITT'S LYMPHOMA (Fig. 2-5)

This is a **B**-cell lymphoma, that is considered a small, **non**-cleaved cell lymphoma and is endemic in Africa. This has a *High* grade classification in Working formulation. Burkitt's lymphoma occurs as a result of t**(8;14)** translocation. There is an increased expression of **c-*myc*** proto-oncogene. It is associated with Epstein-Barr Virus (**EBV**). Burkitt's lymphoma is derived from *B-lymphocytes* (considered of a **B**-cell origin).

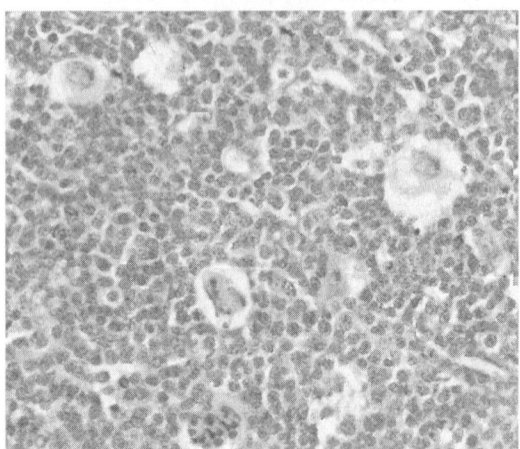

Figure 2-5 Burkitt's lymphoma. This lymphoblastic lymphoma is associated with Epstein-Barr virus, and t(8;14) which activates c-*myc* oncogene. Notice the large macrophages which give the histology slide of the lymphoma a "starry sky" appearance. (For color version see Color Plate 3.)

LYMPHOBLASTIC LYMPHOMA

This is a **T**-cell lymphoma that may present as a *mediastinal mass* in a child with acute leukemia. Lymphoblastic lymphomas make up approximately 40 percent of all childhood lymphomas. It is associated with T-cell ALL, and is considered to be a *very* aggressive lymphoma.

LEUKEMIA

Leukemia is a proliferation of the *leukocytes*. Leukemias are either *acute* (blast cells) or *chronic*. Causes of leukemia include: viruses, radiation, chromosomal abnormalities (like Philadelphia chromosome and Trisomy 21). Leukemia is the most common malignancy in children.

ACUTE MYELOBLASTIC LEUKEMIA (AML)
AML may present in a *young* person with fatigue, bruising, nosebleeding, and a non-palpable spleen. In the laboratory, this is a *normo*cytic *normo*chromic anemia without polychromasia. Furthermore, you will see *blast cells* in the peripheral blood smear. *Myeloperoxidase staining* differentiates AML from ALL.

ACUTE LYMPHOBLASTIC LEUKEMIA (ALL)
ALL has the best prognosis of the acute leukemias. It has an increased incidence during childhood. ALL is usually a non-T, non-B, **calla** + leukemia. Because of the good prognosis, you can expect a prolonged survival with proper therapy. In the laboratory, ALL may present with thrombocytopenia. B-ALL shows an increased expression of **c-*myc*** oncogene.

CHRONIC MYELOCYTIC LEUKEMIA (CML)
CML is also known as Chronic Myeloid Leukemia and Chronic Granulocytic Leukemia and is common in the "middle-aged, 35- to 50-year-olds." CML is associated with a reciprocal translocation at chromosomes **9** and **22** or **t(9;22)**, forming what is known as the *Philadelphia chromosome*. This creates a hybrid oncogene, **bcr-abl**, which is responsible for the pathology in a tyrosine kinase protein causing CML. In the laboratory, we will find: *leukocytosis*, a decreased leukocyte alkaline phosphatase activity, and the Philadelphia chromosome in the precursor cells. Chronic granulocytic leukemia is associated with: splenomegaly, blast crisis (transformation into *acute* leukemia), and increased number of basophils.

CHRONIC LYMPHOCYTIC LEUKEMIA (CLL)
CLL is usually of a **B**-cell origin and is common in *elderly* men (remember, CLL as "chronic, older life"). The leukemic cells infiltrate bone marrow, nodes, and other organs. They can**not** differentiate into plasma cells; therefore, they can**not** form antibodies. In the laboratory, we will find: *smudge cells* in the peripheral blood smear with increased leukemic cells. It is associated with *warm*-antibody autoimmune hemolytic anemia, lymphadenopathy, and hepatosplenomegaly. With treatment, individuals with CLL may survive another 7 years.

CHRONIC GRANULOMATOUS INFLAMMATION

Well-circumscribed aggregates of mononuclear phagocytes and lymphocytes. May or may not have multinucleated giant cells.

ANEMIA

Anemia is a decrease in the hemoglobin and/or red blood cells. It can occur because of excessive use of blood, or a decrease in the production of blood. The *reticulocyte count* will increase or decrease respectively. Anemia presents as: skin pallor, increased heart rate, dizziness, and fatigue. It can be due to: hemorrhage (blood loss), hemolysis, congenital hemolytic anemia (hemoglobinopathies—sickle cell anemia), acquired hemolytic anemias (autoimmune disease), nutritional iron, vitamin B_{12} or folate deficiency.

If a patient is presented with *hypochromic microcytic anemia*, the **serum iron** is *decreased* and the **total iron binding capacity** (TIBC) is *increased*—since the iron is decreased and there are many binding sites available. Yet, there is an *increase* in the serum ferritin and stainable hemosiderin in a bone marrow aspiration. Therefore, the most likely diagnosis is *Iron Deficiency Anemia*. Evaluation of the marrow *hemosiderin* (not ferritin) is a sensitive measure of iron deficiency. Rheumatoid arthritis (RA) usually presents with anti-IgG antibodies.

Iron deficiency anemia is associated with: decreased serum iron, decreased hematocrit and red cell count, decreased marrow hemosiderin (low pigment, iron hemoglobin), decreased serum ferritin (low stores of iron), and *increased* TIBC (*increased* **t**otal **i**ron **b**inding **c**apacity since less iron). It is considered a **hypo**chromic, **micro**cytic anemia.

Again, with a patient who looks anemic, and the results from the lab show a hypochromic microcytic anemia, take notice if the serum iron decreased and TIBC is increased. Next, you should do x-ray visualization studies of the upper and lower GI tract for a GI source of bleeding.

Pernicious Anemia
Megaloblastic anemia due to *intrinsic factor deficiency*. Pernicious anemia is associated with: stomatitis, achlorhydria, glossitis, subacute combined (posterolateral) degeneration—CNS degeneration, and anti-intrinsic factor antibodies.

Sickle Cell Anemia
This hemolytic anemia involves homozygous expression of the **hemoglobin S** gene. It is associated with: African-*American* inheritance, severe lifelong anemia, non-healing leg ulcers, aplastic crisis, *recurrent abdominal and chest pain*, unconjugated hyperbilirubinemia, autosplenectomy (NOT splenomegaly), erythrocyte polychromasia, and reticulocytosis. In areas with malaria, like Africa, the hemoglobin S gene allows resistance to a malarial infection. The S results from a *point* mutation at the hemoglobin gene codon 6 substituting **Valine** for glutamic acid.

Microinfarcts (vasoocclusive phenomena) lead to *painful crisis*, and the **ma**croinfarcts will lead to *organ damage*.

SICKLE CELL TRAIT
This is the *heterozygous* form of the hemoglobin S gene. These patients usually carry the gene, and do NOT have clinical symptoms.

HEMOGLOBIN C DISORDERS
This results from a defect in the hemoglobin gene, and is also predominantly found among African-Americans. It presents as: hemolytic anemia, *splenomegaly*, with *target cells*.

G6PD DEFICIENCY
Glucose-6-phosphodehydrogenase deficiency is associated with drug sensitivity. Hemolysis may be initiated from reducing agents or drugs (antimalarials, sulfonamides) if an individual is deficient in G6PD. These patients should avoid these drugs that may induce hemolysis.

β-THALASSEMIA
β-Thalassemia results from gene defects in the: promotor region, introns, and the coding region—all leading to the premature stop codon formation (NOT from defects in the coding region leading to amino acid substitutions—which occurs in sickle cell anemia).

DIRECT COOMBS' TEST
This test is used in diagnosing *immune* (versus non-immune) red blood cell hemolysis. For example, it is used in a young patient with *hemolytic anemia*, or with hereditary spherocytosis (spherocytes in the peripheral blood smear). *Warm*-antibody hemolytic anemias include: idiopathic anemias, CLL, SLE, and from drug reactions (penicillin, quinidine, sulfonamides, etc.). *Cold*-antibody hemolytic anemias include: infections from mycoplasma, EBV, and syphilis. Therefore, if the cbc from the lab indicates: *anemia* and reticulocytes and the peripheral smear shows *microspherocytes*; then, the additional lab test needed is: Direct Coombs' Test.

HEMOSIDERIN
Hemosiderin is a hemoglobin *pigment* that contains *ferritin* (the storage form of iron). Hemosiderin is found in hepatocytes, Kupffer cells, and bile duct epithelium in Hemosiderosis with: diabetes, increased hepatocellular carcinoma, and abnormal pigmentation of skin (NOT in Kayser-Fleischer ring). *Prussian blue* reaction detects hemosiderin.

HEREDITARY SPHEROCYTOSIS
Hereditary spherocytosis is associated with: polychromatophilic red cells in a peripheral smear, splenomegaly, pigment gall stones, and *increased* MCHC (mean corpuscular hemoglobin concentration) (but, NOT bilirubinemia).

RH-MEDIATED HEMOLYTIC DISEASE OF THE NEWBORN

This hemolytic disease is seen when the following occurs:

Infant = **Rh Positive** and the direct Coombs' test is *positive*
Mother = **Rh Negative** and the direct Coombs' test is *positive*

(Remember, the direct Coombs' test tells us that it is an immune hemolysis.)

CHRONIC ISCHEMIA

Chronic ischemia produces degenerative changes and atrophy, and is frequently caused by stenosis of arteries (by atherosclerosis). It may cause *pain* in the area of ischemia, and affects metabolically active cells. Cell ischemia results in: decreased oxidative phosphorylation, decreased cell membrane ATPase activity, inability to form ATP, and *increased* intracellular *sodium*.

CELLULAR ANOXIA

Anoxia is associated with impaired oxidative phosphorylation, release of enzymes into the blood, a decrease in the ATP reserve, and a change to **an**aerobic glycolysis. Mitochondria are the cellular organelle affected earliest by anoxia.

Sequence of oxygen-dependent system of bacterial killing

$$O_2 \rightarrow O_2^- \rightarrow H_2O_2 \rightarrow Cl_2O_2^-$$

GRANULOMA

A granuloma is an aggregation of *macrophages* transformed into epithelial-like cells. A lesion is a *granuloma* if it has modified monocytes. Examples include: **non**-caseating *sarcoid* epithelioid granulomas, versus *tuberculous* caseous granulomas. Granulomatous response is seen with: Tuberculosis, schistosomiasis, cat-scratch disease, and coccidioidomycosis.

CHRONIC GRANULOMATOUS DISEASE OF CHILDHOOD

Impaired killing of *catalase positive* microorganisms, like *Staphylococcus aureus*. Deficiency of leukocyte membrane **NADPH oxidase**. Impaired leukocyte production of oxygen, H_2O_2, and Cl_2O_2. (NOT decreased leukocyte SOD, NOT decreased leukocyte myeloperoxidase, and NOT impaired killing of catalase *negative* organisms.)

AMYLOIDOSIS

This is associated with rheumatoid arthritis and multiple myeloma. In primary amyloidosis, amyloid *fibrils* are biochemically similar to immunoglobulin *light* chains. Amyloid is made of fibrils with a beta-pleated sheet configuration on x-ray crystallography.

Amyloid types include:

- **AL** or amyloid light chain protein: found in B-cell diseases like multiple myeloma and considered a *primary* amyloidosis. AL is the most common type of amyloid.
- **AA** or amyloid-associated protein: found in inflammatory states like rhematoid arthritis and considered a secondary or reactive amyloidosis.
- *Transthyretin:* hereditary, and found in familial polyneuropathy and aging.
- β_2-*amyloid* (A_4) *protein:* found in Alzheimer's plaques.
- β_2-*microglobulin:* found in long-term hemodialysis.

CONNECTIVE TISSUE DISEASES

SJÖGREN'S SYNDROME
Consider Sjögren's syndrome in a female with an autoimmune disease such as rheumatoid arthritis, with enlarged bilateral parotid glands, dryness of mouth *(xerostomia)* and eyes *(keratoconjunctivitis sicca)*, hypergammaglobulinemia, ANA specific for anti-**SS-A** and -**SS-B**, and lymphocytic infiltration of the parotid and lacrimal glands.

SYSTEMIC LUPUS ERYTHEMATOSUS (SLE)
SLE is considered a connective tissue disease that usually affects women. It affects many organ systems, but mainly the kidneys. *(See SLE for further discussion).* On laboratory exam, the glomerular changes appear as *wire loops* and thickened basement membranes, and most patients are *ANA positive*, with a specific Smith (**Sm**) antigen reaction.

RAYNAUD'S PHENOMENON
This is always *secondary* to another disorder (like SLE or scleroderma). It is aggravated by cold temperatures. (Raynaud's *Disease* is a *disease* of recurrent vasospasm of the small arteries and arterioles, and appears as *cyanosis*.)

SCLERODERMA
This is also known as progressive systemic sclerosis. It is fibrosis that occurs in the skin, GI, and other organs. It is associated with: ANA anti-**Scl-70**, sclerodactyly (claw-like hand), pulmonary fibrosis, and is part of the **CREST** Syndrome. (Remember, CREST stands for **C**alcinosis, **R**aynaud's phenomenon, **E**sophageal dysfunction, **S**clerodactyly, and **T**elangiectasia.)

POLYARTERITIS NODOSA
This is a vasculitis (fibrinous necrosis) that affects the small and medium arteries. It may be caused by medications (i.e., penicillin) and is associated with: hypertension, splenomegaly, abdominal pain, and dyspnea.

EXUDATES

This is edema fluid from *inflammation*. Purulent exudate is composed of "pus" fluid, fibrin, **neutrophils**, necrotic debris, pathogenic organisms, or it may be sterile. Exudates are found in the extravascular location, with an increased specific gravity > 1.018. There is an increased protein concentration, and the presence of leucocytes. On lab examination look for: protein > 4, glucose < 50, increased white blood cell count, and specific gravity > 1.018.

TRANSUDATES

This is **non**inflammatory edema fluid that has a *decreased* protein concentration, and a low white blood cell count. Specific gravity is less than 1.012. *Specific gravity* of serous fluids is proportional to the *protein concentration*.

GRANULATION TISSUE

Has primarily fibroblasts and endothelial cells. Granulation tissue is more abundant in healing by *second* intention than first. (Granulation tissue is NOT an essential component of granulomatous inflammation.)

ACID-BASE DISTURBANCES
Metabolic Acidosis and Alkalosis

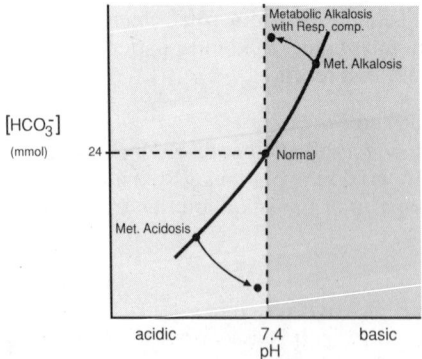

METABOLIC ACIDOSIS

During metabolic acidosis, you may find a decrease in pH (acidosis), a decrease in pCO_2, and a decrease in HCO_3^-. Causes of metabolic acidosis include: GI loss of bicarbonate secondary to diarrhea, *renal loss* of bicarbonate due to renal tubular acidosis, and renal dysfunction due to pyelonephritis and obstruction. Furthermore, it can be due to: increased acid production (secondary to DKA, lactic acidosis), failure to excrete the acid (acute or chronic renal failure), inborn errors of metabolism, and ingestion of ethylene glycol, methanol or acids (drugs). Compensation for metabolic acidosis is achieved by increasing the ventilation rate.

To learn the changes in pH, pCO_2, and HCO_3^-, learn that in *metabolic* acidosis all of the signs are usually "<". Therefore, start with *acidosis* or pH is **< 7.4**, then, pCO_2 is **< 40**, and HCO_3^- is **< 24**.
[Remember, < < <]
Use this technique to simplify learning all of the acid-base disturbances.

METABOLIC ALKALOSIS
During metabolic alkalosis, you may find an *increase* in pH (alkalosis), an increase in pCO_2, and an increase in HCO_3^-.
[Remember, > > >]
This results from increased bicarbonate ingestion, loss of acid (vomiting). Compensated metabolic alkalosis: Decreased pO_2, increased pCO_2, pH, and bicarbonate concentration. Compensation of *metabolic* alkalosis is by respiratory *hypoventilation* (which increases the pCO_2). Respiratory compensation may be *partial* (near to the normal pH of 7.4), because it is less efficient in compensating than the kidneys.

RESPIRATORY ACIDOSIS
During respiratory acidosis, you may find a *decrease* in pH (acidosis), increase in pCO_2, and increased HCO_3^-.
[Remember, < > >]
Compensation of *respiratory* acidosis is by *renal* excretion of the acid and reabsorption of the bicarbonate.

Respiratory Acidosis and Alkalosis

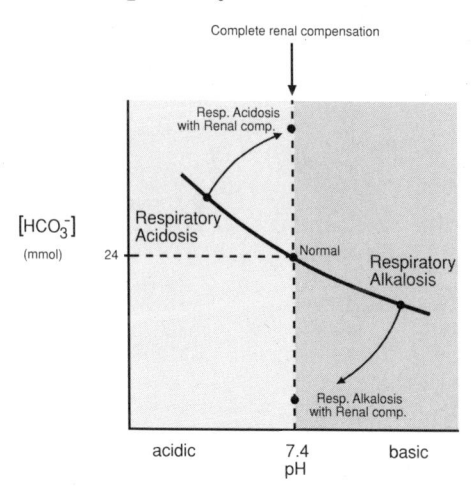

Respiratory Alkalosis

During respiratory alkalosis, you may find an *increased* pH (alkalosis), and a decreased pCO$_2$ and bicarbonate.

[Remember, < > >]

Compensation of *respiratory* alkalosis is by *renal* excretion of *bicarbonate*. Renal compensation is usually *complete* (to pH of 7.4). Respiratory alkalosis occurs during anxiety (increased breathing) and at *high altitudes*.

Acid-Base Balance

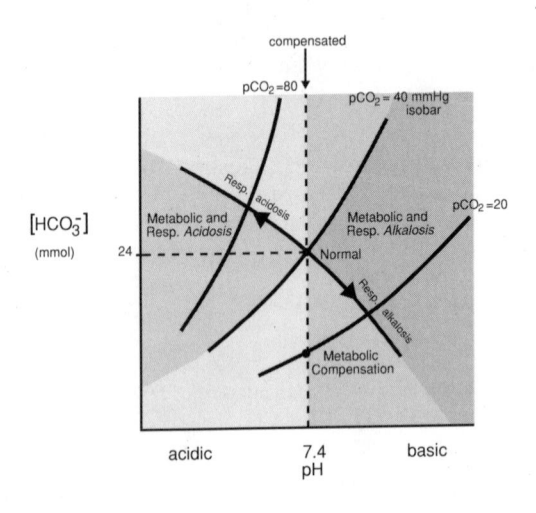

Anion Gap

The anion gap is *increased* in these acid-base disturbances: diabetic ketoacidosis, lactic acidosis, and severe renal disease (but, NOT in renal tubular acidosis).

Cardiovascular 3

MYOCARDIAL INFARCTION (MI)

This is a major cause of death, and may present with arrhythmias and increased myocardial enzymes. Increased pathogenicity with: coronary atherosclerosis and increased oxygen demand on the myocardium. Myocardial infarction complications include: constructive pericarditis, fibrinous pericarditis, hemopericardium with tamponade, ventricular aneurysm, myocardial rupture, and mural thrombosis. Heart enzymes peak in the following order: CPK (1 day), AST (1 to 2 days) and then, LDH (2 to 3 days). CPK = creatine phosphokinase; AST = aspartate aminotransferase; LDH = lactate dehydrogenase.

Collagen deposition indicates that the MI has been there for a *minimum of 2 weeks*.

The *Left* Anterior Descending coronary artery (LAD) is the coronary artery that is usually thrombosed as a cause of a myocardial infarction.

CREATINE KINASE

The CPK level is useful in diagnosing a patient suspected of having a myocardial infarct (MI). If one week has passed after a myocardial infarct, and the patient develops chest pains, changes in EKG, and *increased* levels of this enzyme, then you should suspect that the person is having a *second* infarct. CK-**MB** is the *myocardial* creatine kinase isoenzyme that is more specific for the cardiac muscle.

RHEUMATIC FEVER

This is a multisystem disorder that is caused 1–4 *weeks* after an infection with group **A** β-*hemolytic strep*. Acute stage shows chorea and a recent streptococcus pharyngitis. Therefore, increased titer for antistreptolysin **O**. There may be a positive throat culture for group A β-*hemolytic streptococcus* (NOT positive for rheumatic factor, nor *Strep. viridans*). It is associated with *Aschoff body*, an area of myocardial inflammation and multi-nucleated giant cells. Furthermore, *pancarditis* (pericardium, myocardium, and endocardium) may occur. It is also associated with: fever, increased sed rate, arthritis, and skin lesions. *Endocarditis* is the most serious consequence of acute rheumatic fever.

RHEUMATIC HEART DISEASE

This may occur following rheumatic endocarditis as a result of fibrotic changes and calcification. The valve most frequently involved is the *mitral valve*, then the aortic valve. Rheumatic heart disease is the most common cause of **mitral stenosis**.

INFECTIVE ENDOCARDITIS

This is caused by bacterial or infected endocardium that affects the valve surface. *Right*-sided valve (tricuspid) endocarditis is commonly associated with *drug addicts*. The lumpy, easily detachable *vegetations* contain many bacteria and inflammatory cells that may fragment and cause embolization and infarcts to another part of the body (and the brain) (Fig. 3-1).

ACUTE ENDOCARDITIS
This is associated with *Staph. aureus*.

SUBACUTE (BACTERIAL) ENDOCARDITIS
This is associated with *Strep. viridans*. There is an increased incidence of infective endocarditis involving the *tricuspid valve* in intravenous *drug addicts*.

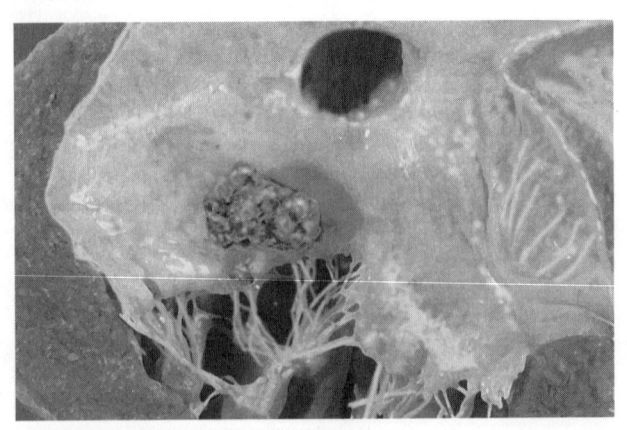

Figure 3-1 Vegetations of mitral valve. Heart valves may form *vegetations*, as in Libman-Sacks endocarditis of an SLE patient or the vegetations may be infective with bacteria and detach—which may occur in IV-drug addicts or after heart surgery. (For color version see Color Plate 4.)

LIBMAN-SACKS ENDOCARDITIS

This endocarditis is associated with SLE (systemic lupus erythematosus). It is NOT associated with carcinoid syndrome, acute rheumatic fever, nor congestive cardiomyopathy.

HYPERTENSION

Hypertension is usually idiopathic (of an unknown cause). Surgically correctable causes of hypertension are: renal artery stenosis, adrenal cortical tumors originating from the zona glomerulosa cells, adrenal medullary tumors, renal tumors originating from juxtaglomerular cells.

A secondary form of pulmonary hypertension is seen with: scleroderma, Tetralogy of Fallot, pulmonary emboli, and chronic hypoxia (NOT tricuspid stenosis).

MALIGNANT HYPERTENSION
Associated with *papilledema*.

SECONDARY HYPERTENSION
Secondary hypertension is caused by: renal artery stenosis, adrenal cortical adenoma, and chronic pyelonephritis (NOT lipoid nephrosis).

PORTAL HYPERTENSION
It is a cause of ascites, esophageal varices, splenomegaly, and portosystemic shunting of toxic products.

RIGHT *VENTRICULAR* DIASTOLIC *PRESSURE*

Direction of shunting at a ventricular septal defect.

MYXOMA

Most common heart tumor.

ATRIAL SEPTAL DEFECT (ASD)

Incomplete separation of the atria. The majority of ASDs are *ostium secundum defects*. This causes a pressure gradient from the left to the *right* atrium. ASD should be corrected surgically before the development of *pulmonary hypertension*.

LUTEMBACHER'S SYNDROME
Atrial septal defect (ostium secundum defect—incomplete closure at the fossa ovalis) and acquired mitral stenosis.

VENTRICULAR SEPTAL DEFECT (VSD)

This is the most frequent congenital heart disease. It is an abnormal opening at the ventricular septum. Therefore, blood will shunt from the left to the *right* ventricle.

TETRALOGY OF FALLOT

This is a right to *left* shunt. This causes cyanosis, *clubbing of the fingers*, and dyspnea. Look for:

1. *Overriding* aorta,
2. *Ventricular* septal defect (VSD),
3. *Pulmonic* stenosis,
4. *Right* ventricular hypertrophy.

(NOT aortic stenosis, nor left ventricular hypertrophy)

CONGESTIVE HEART FAILURE

This is failure of the left and/or right ventricle.

LEFT-SIDED HEART FAILURE

An MI, hypertension, valve disease, and myocarditis are a few causes of *left*-sided heart failure. This CHF is associated with: dyspnea, orthopnea (pulmonary edema), and anoxia (Fig. 3-2).

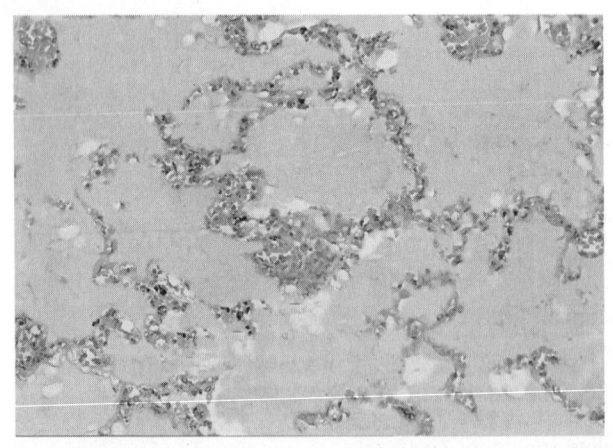

Figure 3-2 Pulmonary edema. Left-sided heart failure may result in edema. The lung alveoli are nearly filled with fluid. Leads to poor lung perfusion and increased systemic venous pressure (engorged jugular vein). (For color version see Color Plate 5.)

RIGHT-SIDED HEART FAILURE

Pulmonary hypertension (from lung disease), mitral stenosis, and *tricuspid/ pulmonary* valve disease are a few causes of *right*-sided CHF. It is associated with: hepatosplenomegaly causing a "nutmeg liver" or congested liver, and ascites (Fig. 3-3).

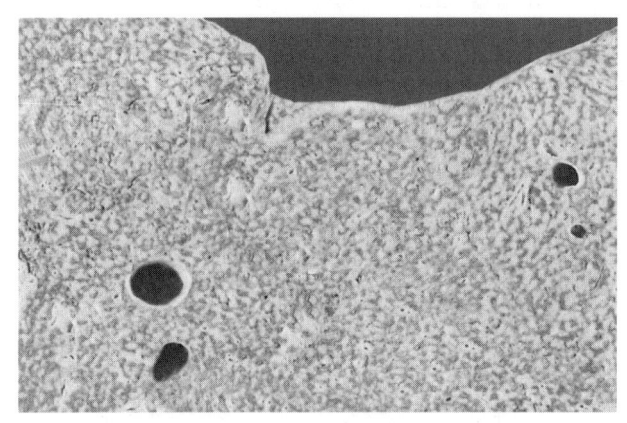

Figure 3-3 Congested liver. Right-heart failure causes an increased IVC pressure, which increases venous pressure in the liver. This causes the liver to "congest" with blood (*dark areas*), and become pale in periportal areas. Appears like a "*nutmeg* liver." (For color version see Color Plate 6.)

COR PULMONALE

This is also known as *pulmonary heart disease*. Cor pulmonale results in *right*-sided hypertension, *right* ventricular dilatation (which leads to tricuspid regurgitation), and hypertrophy that is secondary to pulmonary hypertension. It is caused by disorders of the lung, like COPD and bronchitis.

DISSECTING AORTIC ANEURYSM

Consider a dissecting aortic aneurysm in a 45-year-old with sudden severe tearing chest pain *radiating* downward and to the *back*. This is a common cause of death in Marfan's Syndrome patients.

SEVERE ATHEROSCLEROSIS

Complications include: *abdominal* aortic aneurysm (NOT a *dissecting* aortic aneurysm), coronary and cerebral artery thrombosis.

TAKAYASU'S ARTERITIS

This arteritis (inflammatory disease of the arteries) most commonly affects arteries coming from the *aortic arch*. It is considered the *pulseless disease*, and is associated with weak *upper* extremity pulses and increased pressure in the *lower* extremities.

EMBOLISM

Venous emboli occur from *thrombi* within the deep veins of the legs. *Paradoxical* embolism can occur from an atrial or ventricular septal defect. If a patient dies and doesn't show any gross abnormalities, consider a *Fat* embolism. *Arterial* embolism occurs commonly at sites like the kidneys, spleen, brain, and lower legs. *Pulmonary* emboli occur most commonly from the source: *deep saphenous vein* (Fig. 3-4). An embolus that enters one of the vessels of circle of Willis is most likely from the *pulmonary artery*. A *paradoxical embolism* passes from the *right* to the *left* cardiac circulation. Predisposition to deep vein thrombosis (DVT) includes the following clinical presentations: immobility, post-op patient, pregnancy, and trauma.

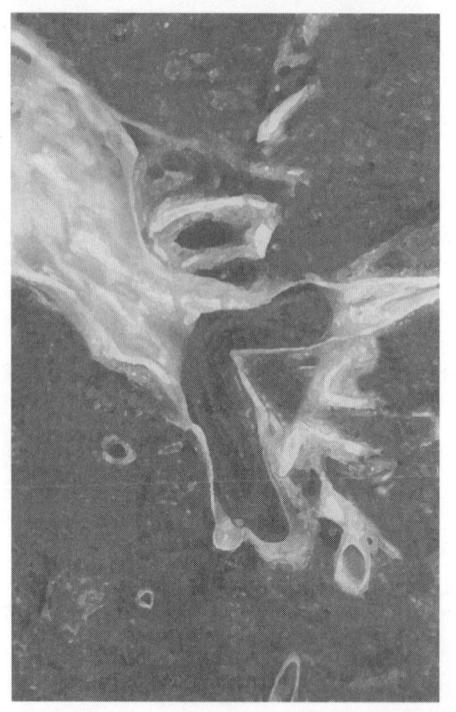

Figure 3-4 Pulmonary thromboembolism. Results from embolization (major origin/cause = deep vein thrombosis). The thromboembolus blocks the pulmonary artery. Leads to ischemia of the lung, and may lead to cardiovascular collapse, chest pain, and death. (For color version see Color Plate 7.)

BROWN ATROPHY OF HEART

Decreased size of myocardial cells (NOT number), accumulation of lipofuscin (NOT homogentisic acid).

SHOCK

Shock affects many organ systems, including the cardiac, pulmonary, hepatic, and renal tissues (but, NOT the muscular system). Acute circulatory shock presents as: cold, clammy skin, feeling weak, having a rapid pulse, pallor, and hypotension.

SEPTIC SHOCK

A decrease in blood pressure and other medical effects as a result of gram-negative, aerobic rods, caused by endotoxins. In burn victims it is usually caused by *Pseudomonas aeruginosa*.

ANTEMORTEM THROMBUS

The antemortem thrombus (blood clot) forms *before* death. It includes the formation of Lines of Zahn, uniform platelets and fibrin in the clot. It involves the endothelium, recanalization, and *adherence* to the vessel wall.

POSTMORTEM CLOT

Will show "chicken fat" and "currant jelly" appearance.

Gastrointestinal 4

PANCREAS, GALL BLADDER, AND LIVER

EXOCRINE PANCREAS
Deficient function of the exocrine pancreas may lead to: fatty liver, nyctalopia, xeropthalmia, and keratomalacia (NOT megaloblastic anemia, nor diarrhea, dementia, nor death).

PANCREATIC INSUFFICIENCY
Microscopically look for fat-staining globules in the stool specimen from patient with persistent diarrhea, and *normal* D-Xylose absorption.

PANCREATIC ENDOCRINE TUMORS
Need RIA for accurate categorization, it may be associated with PUD (peptic ulcer disease). Pancreatic endocrine tumors are considered *malignant*, and usually there is NO palpable mass.

PANCREATIC *DUCTAL* CELLS
Occurs in cystic fibrosis, because of a defective gene in these cells of the pancreas.

PANCREATIC CARCINOMA
Pancreatic carcinoma is associated with: *hemostatic abnormalities*, jaundice, migratory thrombophlebitis, back pain, and diabetes mellitus.

PANCREATITIS
The most common predisposing factors of pancreatitis are: 1. Alcoholism, 2. Trauma, and 3. Gallstones.

IDIOPATHIC HEMOCHROMATOSIS (Fig. 4-1)
This is a familial disorder of increased *iron absorption* (by the intestine). Look for the triad of: hyperglycemia (diabetes mellitus), bronzing of the skin (hyperpigmentation), and cirrhosis of the liver. The pigmentation arises due to

increased *hemosiderin* and *melanin* deposits. On lab examination, you will find an increased serum *iron* and *decreased* TIBC. (*Secondary* hemochromatosis results *secondary to iron overload*.)

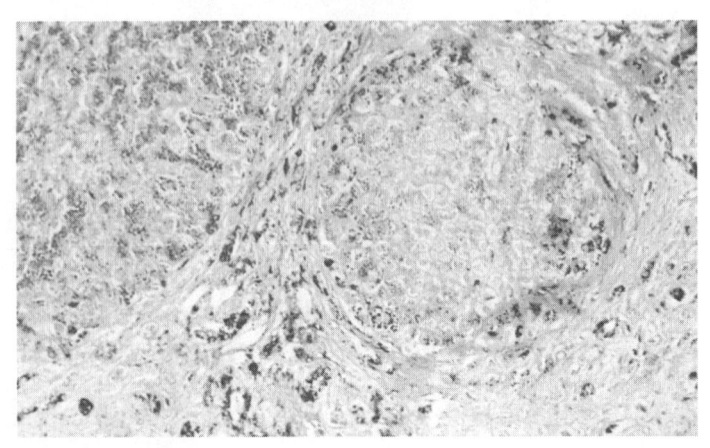

Figure 4-1 Hemochromatosis. Inherited disease (familial) of iron absorption and pigmentation. GI tract increases intake of iron (dietary intake is normal). Toxic iron is stored in the liver, heart, and skin (bronze diabetes). Triad: cirrhosis, diabetes mellitus, increased skin pigmentation. (For color version see Color Plate 8.)

CARCINOMA OF THE GALLBLADDER
Frequent among Native American Indian ancestry.

CARCINOMAS OF EXTRAHEPATIC BILE DUCTS
Arise in a background of sclerosing cholangitis.

GALLSTONES (CHOLELITHIASIS)
Gallstones are VERY COMMON and are seen with: acute and chronic cholecystitis, adenocarcinoma of the gallbladder, and hemolytic anemia. Cholesterol gallstones increase with age, in females, obesity, high-caloric diet, and with drugs like clofibrate. (Remember, the five f's for gallstone risk are: Fat, Fair, Fertile, Female, and Forty.) The GI problems, cirrhosis, and liver fluke infection of the biliary tract can also create gallstones. Stones that pass and obstruct the common bile duct can cause *colic pain*, infection, and damage to the liver. Ultrasonography and cholecystography are used to recognize the stones.

PIGMENT STONES OF BILIARY TRACT
Calcium bilirubinate, older, hereditary spherocytosis, *E. coli* infection of bile (NOT hyperparathyroidism, not ulcerative colitis).

PRIMARY BILIARY CIRRHOSIS
These individuals test positive for anti-mitochondrial antibodies. It is due to choledocolithiasis.

Hyperbilirubinemia
This is an increased bilirubin (BR) concentration. At levels above 2.0 mg/dl, there will be noticeable skin changes (yellowing—*jaundice*) and scleral yellowing (*icterus*).

Unconjugated hyperbilirubinemia
Increased **un**conjugated bilirubin (conjugated BR level is normal). This is seen in: red blood cell destruction—hemolytic anemia, and decreased bilirubin uptake by the liver—from medications like rifampin, and problems with bilirubin *conjugation*—like Gilbert's syndrome.

Conjugated hyperbilirubinemia
Both conjugated and unconjugated bilirubin are *increased*. It is seen in: liver disease, extrahepatic biliary obstruction.

Cholestasis
This is *jaundice* plus *pruritis*, with an increase in conjugated bilirubin, *bile acids*, alkaline phosphatase, and cholesterol.

Dubin-Johnson Syndrome
This autosomal recessive syndrome is diagnosed by liver biopsy. It results in *conjugated* hyperbilirubinemia and a darkly *pigmented* liver from the presence of brown granules in lysosomes.

Rotor's Syndrome
This is an autosomal recessive trait of chronic **a**symptomatic *conjugated* hyperbilirubinemia, but NO pigmented liver.

Gilbert's Syndrome
This is a chronic, mild **un**conjugated hyperbilirubinemia with jaundice, but otherwise normal individual. This is common in Europeans.

Crigler-Najjar Syndrome
This is a congenital disorder that presents as severe to mild **un**conjugated hyperbilirubinemia, with a decreased or absent uridine diphosphate (UDP)-glucuronyltransferase. Therefore, it cannot conjugate the bilirubin in the liver. It results from the cholestasis or obstructed bile flow. This causes the child to be jaundiced. It is associated with: *kernicterus*—toxic accumulation of bilirubin in the brain.

Urine Bilirubin
This is increased with: hepatocellular disease, and biliary obstruction (NOT with hemolytic anemia, nor Gilbert's disease).

Budd-Chiari Syndrome
This syndrome includes: hepatic vein thrombosis with increased thrombotic events like polycythemia vera, pregnancy, oral contraceptives, and cancer.

Fatty change in liver
Fatty change is caused by: increased fatty acids to liver, increased hepatic triglyceride synthesis, and decreased secretion of lipoproteins from liver.

Cirrhosis
Cirrhosis of the liver causes fibrocongestive splenomegaly (it does NOT cause primary splenic lymphoma, mononucleosis, nor Gaucher's), and it is associated with α-1 antitrypsin deficiency, and *galactose*-1-uridyl transferase deficiency (NOT *glucuronyl*-transferase, nor phenylalanine-hydroxylase deficiency). The most common cause of micronodular cirrhosis is from excessive *ethanol* use (alcoholism). In *alcoholic* cirrhosis, there is a slight increase of serum AST, ALT, and alkaline phosphatase levels. Patient has jaundiced appearance. Decreased serum albumin. The cirrhotic liver will always have nodules of regenerating hepatocytes, and fibrous bands (NOT fat and increased iron).

Cirrhosis	Associated with
Alcoholic Cirrhosis	Subendothelial fibrosis
Laennec's Cirrhosis	Micronodular cirrhosis Fatty-Yellow liver
Liver Cirrhosis	Esophageal varices

Galactose-1-phosphate uridyl transferase deficiency
This presents as: infantile cirrhosis, cataracts, hypoglycemia, mental retardation, and decreased sugars in urine.

Hepatocellular injury
Injury to the liver will increase the enzyme: SGPT (ALT) (NOT SGOT/AST).

Alcohol abuse
Alcohol abuse is associated with the following: portal vein thrombosis, esophageal carcinoma, elevated creatine phosphokinase (CPK), and subdural hematoma from trauma or "passing out." Chronic alcoholism is also associated with: Mallory bodies and hyaline inclusion bodies.

Acute hepatitis
Acute hepatitis from: viral hepatitis (like HAV), alcoholic hepatitis, chemical hepatitis, ischemia and congestive liver disease, and hepatic biliary obstruction. It results in increased transaminase and bilirubin levels.

Viral hepatitis
The liver enzymes used to assess viral hepatitis are: ALT and AST.

"Carrier state" of hepatitis
Have serum HBsAg, NO HBsAntibody, NO signs of liver disease (NO HAV carrier state). HBeAg persistence means an acute viral replication and infectivity. IgM anti-HBc is the first antibody, and then anti-HBe. IgG then replaces IgM. Lastly, anti-HBs after the window period.

Hepatitis A
HAV is a ssRNA picor**na**virus. It is considered the "infectious hepatitis," and is transmitted by the oral-fecal route (NOT by parenteral transmission). It is self-limiting, and does NOT have a chronic or carrier state. Usually HAV lesions return to normal. The anti-HAV Ig**M** antibody is present in an *acute infection*. The anti-HAV Ig**G** antibody is present after a few months.

Hepatitis B
Hepatitis B virus is a dsDNA hepa**dna**virus. It is considered the "serum hepatitis," and is *sexually* transmitted. Hepatitis B is the only hepatitis virus with DNA polymerase. H**B**V is transmitted by infected serum or saliva *(parenteral transmission)* and causes jaundice. The first viral marker detected is HBsAg which signifies an *active* HBV infection. Antigen is associated with approximately one third the cases of the immune complex disease—polyarteritis nodosa. All of the following are markers of an *active* HBV infection: *increased* HBsAnti*body*, HBV-DNA polymerase, and ALT action; and a *decrease* of HBeAg. HBV is associated with the "ground glass" hepatocytes. IgM anti-HBc is the first antibody to appear, and then anti-HBeAg appears. The *carrier state* of HBV infection may be asymptomatic, have chronic hepatitis, or have cirrhosis.

> **Fulminant hepatitis**
> This is *massive necrosis* of the liver. It is due to liver transplants, viral hepatitis, drugs, and Wilson's disease. The onset to death of the liver occurs in 2 to 3 weeks. It appears as a massive liver involvement and the liver shrinks in size.

> **Chronic hepatitis**
> The *carrier* state has a normal liver, non-specific changes, and chronic active hepatitis that may progress to cirrhosis. Chronic *active* hepatitis can occur from: Hepatitis **B**, Wilson's disease, autoimmune liver damage, Non-A, non-B hepatitis (HCV), and drug-induced damage. (NOT from Hepatitis **A**—remember, **a**cute) The liver appears as a necrotizing and fibrosing liver, and "moth-eaten." Chronic active hepatitis is also associated with: mononuclear portal inflammation, "piecemeal necrosis," and bridging. The best prognosis is with chronic *persistent* hepatitis.

Non-A, non-B hepatitis
Non-A, non-B hepatitis is considered Hepatitis **C**. It is considered the most frequent cause of *parenteral* hepatitis, and is most likely caused by a **DNA** virus. Think of Hepatitis **C** when *drugs* are involved and in autoimmune hepatitis. Viral hepatitis C is the most common cause of *transfusion-related* hepatitis. This virus develops into a *chronic* state.

Hepatitis D
The Delta agent contains naked **RNA** (not DNA). It may cause fulminant hepatitis. The **δ-agent** causes infection if it has HBsAg as an envelope. For this reason, Hepatitis **D** can only be acquired with a Hepatitis **B** infection—HDV needs HBV.

Acute viral hepatitis
Associated with diffuse involvement of lobules, and Councilman-like hyaline bodies (this is NOT considered a fatal hepatitis).

Chemical hepatitis
Drugs (acetaminophen, amanita phalloides) or hepatotoxins (CCl_4) can cause hepatitis (liver damage). The hepatotoxicity includes changes to the liver like: fatty change and cholestasis. It also causes fulminant hepatitis.

Alcoholic hepatitis
Alcoholic hepatitis is associated with the presence of Mallory bodies, and perivenular sclerosis (NOT submassive hepatic necrosis).

Halothane hepatitis
This is often viral-like. It may appear as fulminant hepatic failure. It may have *granuloma formation*, and increased tissue *eosinophilia*.

Primary tumors of the liver
Hepatoblastoma, Cholangiocarcinoma, Angiosarcoma, Hepatocellular carcinoma.

Hepatocellular carcinoma
There is a decreased incidence of *hepatocellular carcinoma* by vaccination for hepatitis B.

Carcinoma spread by blood vessels
Renal cell carcinoma, and Hepatocellular carcinoma (NOT squamous cell carcinoma of the lung, nor ductal carcinoma of breast).

Hemangiosarcoma of liver
With hemangiosarcoma of the liver, consider *occupational exposure* to carcinogens like: *vinyl chloride* (from plastic PVC manufacturing), *arsenic*. Also, consider exposure to *thorotrast* from radiology of this mid-century.

Mallory bodies
Mallory bodies are associated with *alcoholic* hepatitis (NOT in chronic active hepatitis), Wilson's disease, hepatocellular carcinoma, and cholestasis.

Wilson's disease
Wilson's disease is associated with chronic active hepatitis, degeneration of the lenticular nucleus, Mallory bodies and Kayser-Fleischer rings (copper accumulation) (NOT hepatitis C).

SPLEEN

HYPERSPLENISM
Criteria for the diagnosis of hypersplenism include: *splenomegaly*, leukopenia, reversal of changes after splenectomy, and adequate bone marrow activity (NOT portal hypertension). Some hematologic diseases that may lead to splenomegaly: B-cell lymphoma, T-cell lymphoma, agnogenic myeloid metaplasia, and hereditary spherocytosis.

HYPOSPLENISM
There is a risk of hyposplenism from these pathogens: *Streptococcus pneumoniae*, Malaria parasites, and *Haemophilus influenzae* (NOT *Entamoeba histolytica*).

RANULA
Large mucocele of the floor of the mouth.

PAROTID
This gland has the most malignant salivary gland lesions.

PLUMMER-VINSON SYNDROME
Syndrome includes: a hypochromic microcytic anemia (from chronic iron deficiency), esophageal webs, dysphagia, and atrophic glossitis.

ESOPHAGUS

DYSPHAGIA
One of the chief clinical manifestations of: esophageal atresia, achalasia, esophageal carcinoma, and scleroderma (NOT esophageal varices).

CARCINOMA OF THE ESOPHAGUS
Local spread may prevent complete removal. Carcinoma of the esophagus has a *male* predominance. The patient may have a history of Barrett's esophagitis. This cancer is often asymptomatic until late in the disease (NOT usually an adenocarcinoma). Carcinoma of the esophagus has an increased incidence with *tobacco* and *alcohol* use.

MALLORY-WEISS SYNDROME
Longitudinal linear lacerations in the esophageal lumen. The presenting sign is *hematemesis*—which is not seen in Zenker's diverticulum, traction diverticulum, nor achalasia. Dysfunction of the LES and resulting in vomiting. This is seen with *alcoholics*.

Diverticula of the Esophagus
(Outpouchings of esophagus wall layers):

Zenker's diverticulum
Outpouching of the esophagus immediately *above* the *upper* esophageal sphincter (UES).

Epinephric diverticulum
Outpouching of esophagus immediately *below* the *upper* esophageal sphincter (UES).

Traction diverticulum
Outpouching near the midpoint of the esophagus.

Achalasia
Caused by inadequate relaxation of the lower esophageal sphincter (LES)—this area of the esophagus is constricted and the area above is dilated.

STOMACH

Atrophic Chronic Gastritis
This is the most common chronic gastritis.

Linitis Plastica
An indurated stomach caused by infiltrating adenocarcinoma.

Zollinger-Ellison Syndrome
This is caused by a *gastrinoma* that increases the secretion of gastrin, and thus causes hyperplasia of the parietal and chief cells. The increased gastrin and gastric acid leads to multiple peptic ulcers of the duodenum from an increased secretion of HCl. It is a non-beta islet cell tumor of the endocrine pancreas that increases gastrin secretion.

Classic Adult Pernicious Anemia
Megaloblastic anemia is due to intrinsic factor deficiency. The Schilling test has impaired Vitamin B_{12} absorption. It can be corrected by giving *intrinsic factor* (oral vitamin B_{12} is NOT an effective treatment). It is also associated with: subacute combined degeneration of the cord, and total achlorhydria. There is an increased concentration of gastrin.

Peptic Ulcers
Peptic ulcers are mostly found in the first part of the duodenum (both acute and chronic inflammation).

Gastric ulcer
A gastric ulcer is considered a Peptic Ulcer Disease (PUD) of the *stomach*. PUD is caused by exogenous factors and has an increased incidence in smokers. It may first be diagnosed upon hemorrhage. It is an ulcer with superficial fibrinous exudate, causing an acute inflammation, granulation tissue, and fibrosis. (It does NOT display malignant *transformation*.) Consider gastric peptic ulcers if there are *sharply punched out edges* with radiating gastric folds.

Chronic gastritis
Chronic gastritis may develop with no preceding acute episode. Predisposes to *gastric carcinoma*. In fundal (type A) form, there is an *increased* serum *gastrin* level. It may be associated with anti-parietal cell antibodies.

Atrophic gastritis
High serum *gastrin, low* gastric *acid* secretion.

Carcinoma of stomach
Carcinoma of the stomach is *decreasing* in incidence. It is predisposed by chronic gastritis and gastric polyps. Almost all cancers of the stomach are **adeno**carcinomas.

INTESTINE

Duodenal peptic ulcers
These ulcers are mostly on the anterior wall of the first portion of the duodenum. Duodenal ulcers are usually *benign* and do NOT display malignant transformation. Active stage shows areas of acute and chronic inflammation. Increased level of serum pepsinogen I, parietal cell hyperplasia, with an increased HCl secretion. There is a defect in the secretin release, and an increased response to gastrin or histamine. Duodenal peptic ulcers are NOT confined to the mucosa.

Newborn intestinal obstruction
Occurs with: Intestinal atresia, meconium ileus, and imperforate anus. (Does NOT occur with Meckel's diverticulum)

Meconium ileus
Meconium ileus is associated with *cystic fibrosis* (Fig. 4-2). It is a small bowel obstruction found in a newborn child that appears as a *thickened* meconium, *dilated bowel* with a *thickened, greenish* mucous material filling the bowel. Meconium consists of epithelial cells, mucus, and *bile*. This occurs because of the abnormal mucin that increases in the bowel—which leads to bowel obstruction.

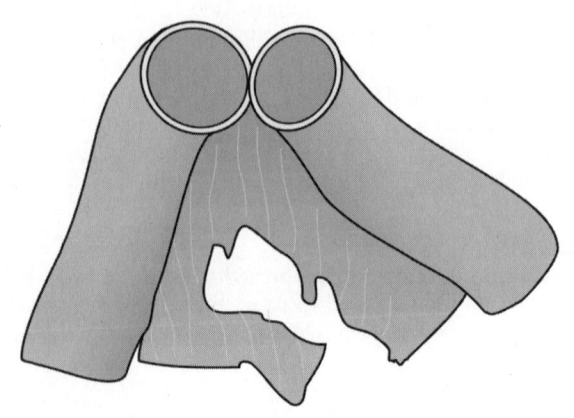

Figure 4-2 Meconium ileus. Meconium ileus is common in cystic fibrosis patients. Viscid mucin forming the thick, green mucus mass and obstruction in the bowel lumen. (For color version see Color Plate 9.)

MECKEL'S DIVERTICULUM
Meckel's diverticulum occurs in the *ileum*.

TOXIC MEGACOLON
This is the most dangerous complication of colitis.

CONGENITAL MEGACOLON
Due to absence of ganglion cells of Meissner and Auerbach plexuses (NOT Chagas' disease).

WHIPPLE'S DISEASE
Whipple's disease is *malabsorption* in the small intestine with systemic problems. It is probably caused by rod-shaped bacteria, and is associated with: polyarthralgias, lymphadenopathy, bacterial, fat malabsorption, increased free fatty acids, and diarrhea. Whipple's disease has serum chylomicrons and fat malabsorption. The bacillary bodies may be in intestinal macrophages (*PAS-positive macrophages* in the lamina propria). Whipple's disease may be complicated by protein-losing enteropathy, and extraintestinal structures. *Histiocytes* are macrophage cells of the small intestine that manifest the characteristic change of Whipple's disease.

CROHN'S DISEASE
This is a chronic, recurrent inflammatory disease of the entire digestive tract. It consists of *fistula tract* formation and *skip lesions throughout* the GI—unlike co**l**itis, which is inflammation at the **col**on. More complicated fistula than ulcerative colitis. Abnormal results in both stages of Schilling test in patient with megaloblastic anemia. Malabsorption. (It does NOT have a frequent malignant change, nor mucosal involvement.) There is *transmural* inflammation, fistulas between bowel loops, "cobblestone appearance" of

mucosa, "serpentine" ulcers, and fibrosis (it is NOT associated with crypt abscesses, nor pseudopolyps). Treatment includes: corticosteroids, *sulfasalazine*, and metronidazole. It may require surgery for obstructions or complications.

ULCERATIVE COLITIS
This chronic inflammatory bowel disease presents as: crypt abscesses, pseudopolyps, superficial *non*-transmural (mucosal) inflammation, increased risk for malignant changes like colonic adenocarcinoma, and toxic megacolon. (It does NOT have granuloma formation nor skip lesions.)

PSEUDOMEMBRANOUS COLITIS
This condition is associated with long-term antibiotic therapy—it causes serious diarrhea from the extended use of drugs like lincomycin or clindamycin. It can be complicated by perforation and peritonitis. If the patient presents with a mucin-rich membrane over a partially necrotic mucosa, and a history of antibiotic use, consider pseudomembranous enterocolitis. The bacterial overgrowth is *Clostridium difficile*.

CARCINOID SYNDROME
Carcinoid syndrome is associated with right heart failure, tumors with malignant potential, and hepatic metastasis—*ileal carcinoids*. Carcinoid tumors arise from endocrine cells in the GI tract mucosa. The cells are *argyrophilic* or silver staining. It may occur with primary carcinoid of the lung in the absence of hepatic metastasis. Signs and symptoms caused by secretory products of the tumor include: prominent diarrhea, asthma-like wheezing, and paroxysmal *flushing*. The principal mediator (neuroendocrine) is *serotonin* (5-HT). Other neuroendocrine secretions include: calcitonin, bradykinin, substance P, kallikrein, and prostaglandins.

MARASMUS
This is the deficiency of nutrients, especially *protein* **and** *calorie* malnutrition. Usually the patient is less than 1 year old, and lacked the proper breast feeding or nutrition. It appears as: retarded growth, and loss of muscle (protein wasting) and subcutaneous fat.

KWASHIORKOR'S
This is a *protein* deficiency with *adequate* calories. Decreased amount of plasma albumin. The decreased *protein* will result in *edema*. If severe, you will see *decreased* blood levels of: Prothrombin, β-lipoprotein, transferrin, and retinol binding protein. Kwashiorkor is due to severe protein deficiency and presents with: anemia, edema (from hypoalbuminemia), an *enlarged belly*, increased fatty acid synthesis, decreased lipoprotein synthesis (NOT decreased immunoglobulins). An infant in the terminal stages has stool with increased amino acids.

CELIAC DISEASE (CELIAC SPRUE)
Celiac disease is also known as *gluten-sensitive enteropathy*. It is likely an immunologic disorder reacting to *gliadin* (of gluten). Abnormal D-Xylose test

(abnormal absorption). (But, NO biliary obstruction, and NO pancreatic insufficiency.) It is associated with HLA-B8 and Dw/DR3, and DR7. The treatment is a *gluten-free diet*—Beware of wheat!

TROPICAL SPRUE
Occurs in epidemics. Tropical sprue can be treated with folic acid and tetracycline. (It is NOT caused by a reaction to gluten, and is NOT common in the USA.) Enterotoxigenic *E. coli* (ETEC) may be a cause of tropical sprue.

MALABSORPTION OF *UPPER* GI
It is difficult to absorb the vitamins A, D, E, and K, and this may lead to the development of: night blindness and keratomalacia (since vitamin absorption is decreased), osteomalacia (from vitamin D deficiency) and hemorrhagic phenomena (from vitamin K deficiency—NOT Vitamin B_{12} deficiency).

INTESTINAL MALABSORPTION
Consider intestinal malabsorption in an older female with a bone biopsy showing osteoid that *lacks* mineral in the peripheral portions.

CONGENITAL LACTOSE INTOLERANCE
Absence of specific intestinal disaccharidase. It may complicate celiac disease or tropical sprue (lactose intolerance is NOT diagnosed by biopsy).

COLON CANCER
Increased risk with an increased dietary fat, decreased fiber content, bile acids, fecal intestinal flora nitrosamines (carcinogenic).

GUAIAC TEST
If the guaiac test is positive, it is suggestive of occult blood in the stool from an internal bleed. Therefore, do a guaiac test on anyone who is admitted to a hospital, and definitely on a person with a decreased hemoglobin or hematocrit. The source of the anemia may be from a gastrointestinal loss.

ADENOCARCINOMA IN THE *CECUM*
Adenocarcinoma of the *right side* of the colon, rather than the *left side* of the colon (i.e., sigmoid colon), is usually associated with symptoms like weakness and weight loss. This allows for *earlier* diagnosis of *right-sided tumors*, since it is likely to cause an obstruction at an early stage. Adenocarcinoma in the cecum is associated with adenomatous polyps. (It does NOT cause iron deficiency anemia, and is NOT metastatic initially.)

LESIONS OF THE GI TRACT THAT *RARELY* DEVELOP MALIGNANT TRANSFORMATION:
Polyp of Peutz-Jegher's syndrome, and hyperplastic polyp.

LESIONS OF GI TRACT THAT *DEVELOP* MALIGNANT TRANSFORMATION:
Ulcerative colitis, Polyp of Gardner's syndrome, Adenomatous polyp.

CAUSES OF INTESTINAL STRANGULATION
Intussusception and Volvulus (NOT polypoid tumor, NOT bezoar).

Intussusception
This is the movement of a proximal part of the intestine into the distal part. It is usually seen in children (Fig. 4-3).

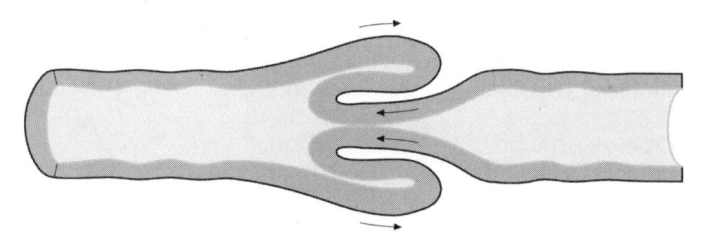

Figure 4-3 Intussusception. (For color version see Color Plate 10.)

Intraabdominal hernia
Necrosis can also occur from strangulation of the intestine in a hernial sac. This results from the pushing out and strangulation of a part of the intestine, and then ischemia and necrosis (Fig. 4-4).

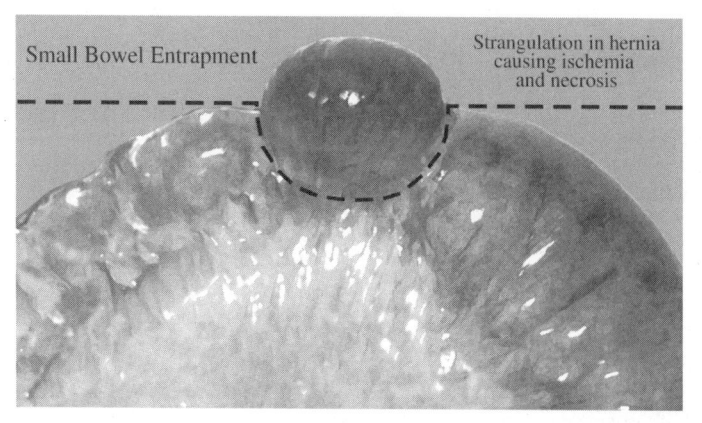

Figure 4-4 Intraabdominal hernia. (For color version see Color Plate 11.)

Volvulus
Volvulus is the *twisting* of a portion of the bowel, with adhesions, and results in venous congestion, ischemia, and necrosis—this is associated with a recent abdominal surgery near the affected intestine. The venous infarction causes congestion of venous blood.

Napkin-ring constriction
This occurs mostly in the *left* colon.

Diverticular disease of the colon
The patient is usually asymptomatic. The lesion is a herniation of the mucosa and submucosa through the muscular layer. It is complicated by bleeding. (These patients do NOT have increased incidence of colon carcinoma.)

Kruckenberg's Tumor
Bilateral metastatic, mucin-producing (signet-ring) cells in the *ovaries* that originate from the *GI tract*.

Transmural Bowel Infarcts
Acute abdomen due to contraceptives, cardiac failure, polycythemia, valvular prosthesis, or arterial thrombosis, and can find gangrene.

Abetalipoproteinemia
Abetalipoproteinemia is associated with: impaired vision and ataxia, bulky stools with steatorrhea, and a normal xylose test. Lipid droplets in villi of jejunum.

Steatorrhea
Check the percentage of fat in a 72-h stool in patients with persistent steatorrhea.

Respiratory 5

PRIMARY PULMONARY HYPERTENSION (IDIOPATHIC)

This increased pulmonary arterial pressure results following an increase in the pulmonary vasculature *resistance*. It is associated with: young women or children, fatigue, progressive dyspnea, respiratory insufficiency, cor pulmonale, atheromatous changes in the larger pulmonary arteries, and finally death.

SECONDARY PULMONARY HYPERTENSION

Usually this pulmonary hypertension occurs *secondary* to: COPD—**c**hronic **o**bstructive **p**ulmonary **d**isease—or interstitial lung disease, *left*-sided heart disease with recurrent pulmonary emboli, or mitral stenosis (NOT lobar pneumonia).

PULMONARY THROMBOEMBOLISM AND INFARCTION

The pulmonary artery may be occluded by thrombosis or from an *embolus*. The embolus usually originated from a lower extremity vein or a pelvic vein. This affects the *venous* system and results in CHF, shock, and sudden death. If the pulmonary artery is affected near the right ventricle this is called a *saddle embolus*. This may be associated with: long bone fractures, immobilization, carcinoma, age, and obesity (see Fig. 3-4).

PHEOCHROMOCYTOMA

Pheochromocytomas will cause an increased peripheral resistance hypertension, palpitations, and perspiration. Remember the "10% rule": Pheochromocytomas are *multiple* in about 10% of patients, *malignant* in 10% of cases, 10% occur in *children*, 10% are *familial*, and they are *extra-adrenal* in about 10% of patients. They are diagnosed by: *increased* epinephrine, metanephrine, normetanephrine, and *vanilylmandelic acid* or VMA (NOT an increased 5-hydroxyindolacetic acid).

GOHN COMPLEX

Tuberculous nodule within the lung with hilar *nodal* involvement.

WEGENER'S GRANULOMATOSIS

Wegener's granulomatosis involves both the respiratory tract and the kidney (renal immunity). The complex vasculitis occurs with granulomatous lesion of the upper and lower respiratory tract.

CYSTIC FIBROSIS

Cystic fibrosis is an *autosomal recessive* disorder common to *Whites* and involves the long arm of chromosome 7. It is an exocrine gland disorder where there is mucus (the thick mucus can obstruct organs like the intestine), and an *increased* sweat *chloride* concentration. It is associated with meconium ileus, steatorrhea, and recurrent respiratory infections. *Staphylococcus aureus*, *Pseudomonas aeruginosa*, and *Pseudomonas cepacia* are the infections to look out for.

BLOODY PLEURAL FLUID

Bloody fluid discharge or cough from the lung is suggestive of trauma, *malignancy*, and tuberculosis (but, NOT pyogenic infection of lung).

INFLAMMATORY LUNG DISORDERS

ACUTE BRONCHITIS
This affects the large bronchi and is usually caused by a cold virus or bacteria. Neutrophils are involved.

CHRONIC BRONCHITIS
Initial symptom is persistent productive cough (with sputum) for at least 3 months in the last 2 years. It occurs as a result of chronic irritation of the airways (i.e., from cigarette smoke) and this increases the mucus production and the number of secondary infections. There is marked hypertrophy of the mucous glands. Atypical metaplasia or dysplasia of bronchial epithelium is often seen. In severe cases, there is obliteration of the lumen of the bronchioles (bronchiolitis obliterans). Cor pulmonale *is* a complication of this.

BACTERIAL PNEUMONIA
Bacterial pneumonia is usually caused by *Streptococcus pneumoniae*. The histology of pneumococcal *lobar* pneumonia will appear as: intra-alveolar neutrophils, red cells, and fibrin. (NOT prominent interstitial inflammatory cell collections with relatively clear alveolar spaces. NOT necrotic tissue, nor abscess formation, and NO fibrosis and scarring.)

VIRAL INTERSTITIAL PNEUMONIA
Viral pneumonia presents as: interstitial mononuclear infiltrates, hyaline membranes, and widening of alveolar septa (NOT a formation of pyogenic abscesses).

ATYPICAL PNEUMONIA
This is usually caused by *Mycoplasma pneumoniae*. It is usually seen in young adults or children. This is an *interstitial* pneumonia, and is "atypical" due to the lack of exudates and consolidation seen with pneumococcal pneumonia.

TUBERCULOSIS
Primary pulmonary tuberculosis is caused by *Mycobacterium tuberculosis*. The original lesion is called the Ghon's lesion. The *Ghon complex* is the initial Ghon's lesion *plus* the affected lymph nodes. Secondary Tuberculosis (Recrudescence) has a preferential involvement of the *apex* of the lung.

LEGIONNAIRE'S DISEASE
This infection is known to occur from air-conditioning systems contaminated by *Legionella pneumopilia* and is more common in the elderly and immunocompromised hosts.

HISTOPLASMOSIS
This is endemic to the Ohio-Mississippi river valley areas. Histoplasmosis may disseminate to the bone marrow, peripheral blood, liver, and the spleen. Tissue granulomatous reactions (calcified granulomas) are very common. Otherwise, the patients are usually asymptomatic.

COCCIDIOIDOMYCOSIS
This is endemic to the San Joaquin Valley (desert region of the Southwestern U.S.).

ASPERGILLOSIS
This is associated with AIDS and immunosuppressed individuals. Microscopically, there are *branching hyphae*. Septic hemorrhagic infarction is most often seen with aspergillosis.

CHRONIC OBSTRUCTIVE PULMONARY DISEASE (COPD)
Emphysema and chronic bronchitis (and asthma) are considered chronic obstructive pulmonary disease. These diseases include increased resistance to air flow because of a chronic expiratory obstruction. In *emphysema*, there are enlarged air spaces and the walls are destroyed. An emphysema patient appears as a "pink puffer." In *panacinar* emphysema, there is an enzyme deficiency of α-*1 antitrypsin*. In *centriacinar* emphysema, the individual is most likely a male, smoker, with a history of chronic bronchitis.

PULMONARY EMPHYSEMA
This is an abnormal dilatation of alveolar spaces. It is damage to the alveolar walls (rupture alveolar walls) associated with environmental air pollution and cigarette

smoking. Eventually, it creates congestive heart failure, and alveolo-capillary block. *Bullous* emphysema is associated with pneumothorax and blebs.

Panacinar emphysema is associated with homozygous α-1 antitrypsin deficiency. *Centriacinar* emphysema is associated with smokers and chronic bronchitis. Emphysema creates *respiratory acidosis* (NOT alkalosis). (It does NOT decrease the resistance to expiration, and there are NO anti-basement membrane antibodies—which are present in Goodpasture's Syndrome.)

Centrilobular emphysema
This emphysema primarily affects the *respiratory bronchioles*. It involves *smokers* and is associated with chronic bronchitis. This is more common than panlobular emphysema.

Panlobular emphysema
Panlobular emphysema is most closely associated with *α-1 antitrypsin deficiency*.

CHRONIC BRONCHITIS
This is the hypersecretion of mucus and a productive cough, usually resulting from smoking.

LUNG TUMORS

Lung tumors that usually have a *central* origin (near the hilum) include: squamous cell carcinoma and small cell carcinoma. *Peripheral* lung tumors include: adenocarcinoma and bronchioloalveolar carcinoma.

HEMARTOMA
This is a large lobular mass of hyaline cartilage with respiratory epithelium.

BRONCHOGENIC CARCINOMAS OF THE LUNG
These cancers make up 90–95% of all lung cancers. If after a lung resection for a bronchogenic carcinoma the patient has profuse generalized bleeding, then, the labs will show: a prolonged prothrombin time and activated partial thromboplastin time, a decreased fibrinogen concentration or prolonged thrombin time, and an increase in fibrin and fibrinogen split products.

1. Small cell carcinoma of the lung (oat cell carcinoma)
Lung carcinoma is associated with: a history of cigarette smoking, production of hormonal active substances. It is the most common cause for ectopic hormone production. This lung cancer has a POOR prognosis, it is the most malignant lung cancer and results in a central or hilar tumor.

2. Squamous cell carcinoma of the lung
Squamous cell carcinoma of the lung is associated with: Males > females, cigarette smoking, and a *central* location near the hilum. It is more com-

mon than adenocarcinoma. Metastasis occurs by lymphatic and hematogenous routes (Fig. 5-1).

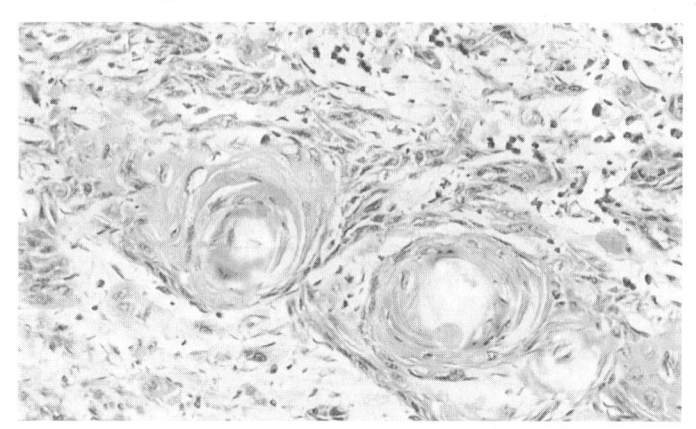

Figure 5-1 Squamous cell carcinoma. Notice the keratin pearls and nests of the malignant squamous epithelium. (For color version see Color Plate 12.)

3. Adenocarcinoma of the lung
Adenocarcinoma of the lung is associated with: a history of *smoking* and old trauma or tuberculosis, usually it is a peripheral mass, gland formation with mucin production. This is a slower growing tumor than squamous cell carcinoma and has a better prognosis.

PARANEOPLASTIC SYNDROMES
These are associated with bronchogenic carcinomas. The hormones released include: ADH (SIADH or Syndrome of Inappropriate ADH secretion), ACTH (Cushing's syndrome), PTH, gonadotropin (gynecomastia), hyperestronism, calcitonin, myasthenia gravis-like syndrome, and serotonin (carcinoid syndrome).

BRONCHIOLOALVEOLAR CARCINOMA
Characteristically this cancer grows along pre-existing alveolar surfaces. It is thought to originate from *type II pneumocytes* and clara cells of the bronchiolar mucosa. The tall columnar mucin-producing cells line the alveolar septa. Adenocarcinoma arising in the terminal bronchioloalveolar regions occur almost always in the lung *periphery*. (This cancer is NOT usually associated with smoking, and does NOT usually have a central location.)

BRONCHIAL CARCINOID
Also known as an *adenoma*. This low grade carcinoma originates from the APUD cells of the bronchus. It is *locally* invasive, but may metastasize. Develop carcinoid syndrome even without hepatic metastasis. Carcinoid syndrome includes: diarrhea, wheezing, flushing, and cyanosis from a bronchial carcinoid. Histologically, it is similar to other argentaffinomas. The treatment is to surgically resect the carcinoid.

SILICOSIS

Inhaled silica causes chronic nodular pulmonary fibrosis. This increases the severity of tuberculosis. It is seen with miners and in sandblasting. The history to look for: coal, gold, and copper mining, and ceramics workers. The coal dust causes a blackening and calcification, and results in collagenous nodules in the lungs.

COAL WORKERS' PNEUMOCONIOSIS

This results in a progressive massive fibrosis and scarring of the lungs—Black Lung Disease. The carbon dust creates a *black sputum*, and macules of coal within the macrophages.

ANTHRACOSIS

Anthracosis is the *harmless* accumulate of city "smog."

SARCOIDOSIS

Sarcoidosis is associated with: enlarged lymph nodes, diffuse interstitial pulmonary infiltrates, multiple *non*-caseating granulomas, Females > Males, and African Americans > whites. To diagnose sarcoidosis you must do a *biopsy* (i.e., the liver or lymph node). It is also associated with the presence of: multinucleated giant cells, Schaumann bodies, and asteroid bodies. Look for multiple organ involvement, **non**-caseating granulomas in a patient with interstitial lung disease and hilar lymphadenopathy (bilateral hilar node enlargement). It has an unknown etiology and no known infectious agent.

MALIGNANT MESOTHELIOMA

This is a *pleural tumor* that results from *occupational exposure* to *asbestos*. Most patients have a history of *asbestos* exposure (approx. 80% of all cases are due to asbestos). Recurrent pleural effusion is a common clinical presentation. This tumor has a very poor prognosis. (Smoking is NOT an important risk factor.)

ASBESTOSIS

Asbestosis is associated with: an increased risk of bronchogenic carcinoma and *malignant mesothelioma*. It appears as asbestos bodies in the lung with fibrous silicates that are curled, serpentine and straight amphiboles. The fibers are ingested by alveolar macrophages and this activates C5a and chemotaxis. Notice the "dumbbell-shaped" asbestos bodies in Fig. 5-2.

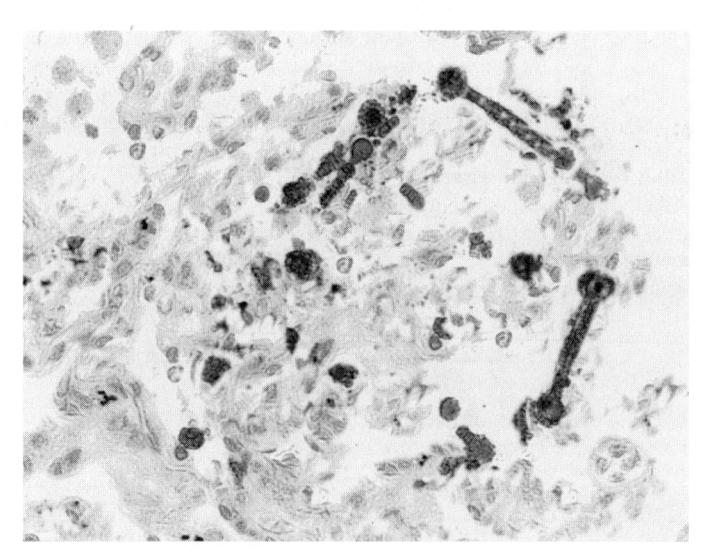

Figure 5-2. Asbestosis. Occupational exposure to the fibrous silicate, asbestos, causes the diffuse interstitial fibrosis. The dumbbell-shaped asbestos bodies form as a result of inhaled asbestos fibers cleared by macrophages, and coated by hemosiderin and glycoproteins. (For a color version see Color Plate 13.)

SINGER'S NODULES

These are benign polyps that are caused by irritation of the vocal cords.

CARCINOMA OF THE LARYNX

Most often *glottic*, then supra or subglottic (poorer prognosis) location. Adenocarcinoma is the most common carcinoma of the larynx, and then squamous cell carcinomas. Males > females. Laryngeal carcinoma is found on the true vocal cords, and may be a *squamous cell* carcinoma in type.

RESPIRATORY DISTRESS SYNDROME (RDS)

RDS presents as respiratory failure that is unresponsive to oxygen therapy. Causes of adult RDS include: inhaled or ingested toxic substances (like smoke), septic shock as a result of severe skin burns or surgery, or from a virus (NOT silicosis). It is initiated by an increased permeability of capillary walls.

Neonatal respiratory distress syndrome (NRDS)
NRDS is also known as *Hyaline membrane disease*. It is a result of the deficiency in pulmonary surfactant. This is associated with: maternal diabetes, a deficiency of *surfactant*, and *prematurity* (<28 weeks, the type II

pneumocytes cannot produce the surfactant; which begins fully at around 35 weeks). In the amniotic fluid, there is a *decreased* Lecithin : Sphingomyelin ratio, which is normally around 2:1. (NOT α-1 antitrypsin deficiency—which is seen with cirrhosis of the liver and emphysema.)

Adult respiratory distress syndrome (ARDS)
ARDS presents as diffuse damage to the alveolar walls by oxygen free radicals, aggregated neutrophils, and decreased surfactant. This results in: atelectasis, and "stiff lungs." Hyaline membrane disease is a decrease in surfactant.

PANCOAST'S SYNDROME

Bronchogenic carcinoma of the *apex* of the lung. This is commonly seen with Horner's syndrome (ptosis, anhidrosis, and miosis).

GOODPASTURE'S SYNDROME

This syndrome presents as a necrotizing, hemorrhagic interstitial *pneumonitis*, and *progressive glomerulonephritis*. It is caused by antibodies against the basement membrane antigens in the *lungs* and *kidneys*.

KARTAGENER'S SYNDROME

This syndrome includes: *Bronchiectasis*, Sinusitis, and *Situs inversus viscera* (internal organs are on the opposite side) (NOT hydrothorax, nor webbed neck).

PLEURITIS

Pleuritis is caused by a small embolus to the lung, and may be seen in a young patient. The two patterns of inflammation of the pleura are: *serofibrinous* and *suppurative* pleuritis.

HYDROTHORAX

This is the accumulation of *transudate* (clear serous fluid) in the pleural cavity.

BRONCHIECTASIS

This lesion destroys the bronchial muscularis and replaces it with a collagenous scar. It is usually *segmental*. It may be either congenital or acquired, but is usually secondary to prolonged or repeated pulmonary infection. Bronchiectasis interferes with bronchial cleansing and allows accumulation within the bronchi of large amounts of sputum not easily raised by coughing or ciliary action.

HYPOXIA

Hypoxia causes cell damage by: losing intracellular potassium, decreased intracellular pH (acidic), *increased* intracellular sodium, and *increased* intracellular water.

LUNG ABSCESS

A lung abscess can occur with: chronic sinusitis, carcinoma, bronchiectasis, and persistent vomiting (NOT from bronchial asthma).

Endocrine 6

PITUITARY AND ADRENAL GLANDS

ADDISON'S DISEASE
Addison's disease is also known as *Primary chronic adrenocortical insufficiency* (or primary adrenal insufficiency). This adrenal cortical hypofunction is usually due to an autoimmune adrenalitis or atrophy. The serum cortisol level is borderline to low, there is an increased ACTH, and decreased *urine* 17-hydroxy corticosteroids. This disease is the result of an idiopathic atrophy of the adrenal gland (adrenal *cortex*), and causes hyperpigmented skin (secondary to increased ACTH), hypotension, nausea, vomiting, weight loss, and fatigue (NOT hypokalemia). If the patient is given ACTH or metyrapone over a few days, the urine 17-hydroxy corticosteroids remain unchanged (it does NOT increase).

MULTIPLE ENDOCRINE NEOPLASIA SYNDROME (MEN TYPE II)
MEN type II**a** is also known as Sipple's Syndrome. This syndrome includes:

1. *Medullary* Thyroid carcinoma,
2. Pheochromocytoma,
3. Parathyroid hyperplasia.
   (NOT a pituitary adenoma)

MEN type II**b** includes the following:

1. *Medullary* Thyroid carcinoma,
2. Pheochromocytoma,
3. Mucosal neuromas.

CONN'S SYNDROME
Conn's Syndrome is also known as *Primary* Hyperaldosteronism. It presents with *low* renin. An increase in aldosterone increases the NaCl reabsorption and decreases the potassium by increasing the K^+ excretion. Think of Conn's

Syndrome when a *hypertensive* patient has labs with: increased sodium and chloride, and decreased potassium (increased sodium absorption and potassium excretion). Normal creatinine, and increased urea and glucose.

SECONDARY HYPERALDOSTERONISM
Increased renin-angiotensin and NaCl retention. Therefore, hypertension results as a complication of hyperaldosteronism. *Secondary* hyperaldosteronism is due to: renal ischemia, edema, or from a renin-neoplasm. In liver disease, this causes ascites.

CUSHING'S *DISEASE*
Cushing's *disease* is the increase in cortical hormones due to an adenoma of the *pituitary*. Usually a *basophilic* adenoma causes *pituitary* Cushing's. A Cushing's disease patient will present with: hypertension, central obesity, glucose intolerance, polycythemia, and *pituitary*-dependent hypercorticism. You can confirm *Pituitary* Cushing's by a dexamethasone suppression test. In Cushing's disease, there will be suppression of both the HIGH and LOW dose dexamethasone tests. The LOW levels of dexamethasone fails to suppress adrenal production of cortisol, but it *does* suppress the *pituitary* production.

[NOTE: If the individual fails to suppress a LOW dose dexamethasone, then it is most likely *Adrenal* Cushing's. If the individual fails to suppress HIGH-dose dexamethasone, then it is most likely *Ectopic* Cushing's.]

CUSHING'S *SYNDROME*
Cushing's *syndrome* is the increase in cortical hormones due to *any* cause (ectopic production of ACTH). This is adrenocortical hyperplasia with increased ACTH. For example, the production of ACTH-like substance by small cell carcinoma of the lung.

PITUITARY ADENOMA
A patient with a pituitary adenoma will have persistent galactorrhea (from hyperprolactinemia), eosinophilic adenoma of pituitary, this causes acromegaly and gigantism (from increased growth hormone), amenorrhea, and carbohydrate intolerance. *Prolactinoma* is the most common pituitary adenoma. Chromo**phobic** cell adenomas are the most common *non*-secretory pituitary adenomas. Non-functional adenomas make up about 10–30% of all pituitary tumors. Anterior pituitary is > *Posterior* pituitary lesions. Remember, the *anterior* pituitary releases growth hormone, prolactin, ACTH, TSH, FSH, and LH. The *posterior* pituitary releases ADH and Oxytocin.

DIABETES INSIPIDUS
This occurs as a result of a *posterior* pituitary *deficiency* of **ADH**. It causes thirst, and may occur secondary to injury to the head and the pituitary area or of idiopathic etiology.

SIADH
This syndrome of inappropriate ADH secretion results as a *posterior* pituitary *increase* in ADH. Ectopic secretion of ADH from a small cell carcinoma of

the lung, pulmonary tuberculosis, or CNS disorder will cause SIADH. Therefore, sodium is decreased, and there is edema.

HYPOPITUITARISM
This may be associated with Sheehan's Syndrome (*anterior* pituitary infarct, pregnancy, shock, and no lactation), chromophobe adenoma of pituitary (nonsecretory), and "empty-sella syndrome" (enlarged sella, but NOT a tumor). It does NOT occur with adrenal Cushing's syndrome. Panhypopituitarism causes Simmond's cachexia.

ANTERIOR PITUITARY INSUFFICIENCY
This results in a decrease of ACTH. Therefore, the serum *cortisol* concentration decreases. In a prolonged ACTH stimulation test, the plasma cortisol level will increase (you may see as much as a three times increase). Anterior pituitary insufficiency occurs from: tumors, sustained hypotension, tuberculous meningitis and septic shock.

APUD TUMORS
APUDomas cause *increased*: ACTH, ADH, PTH, and Serotonin (NOT increased cortisol, nor thyroxin, nor TSH).

HYPERCORTICISM
Hypercorticism can be caused by: pituitary adenomas, adrenal cortical adenoma, and ectopic ACTH production. (NOT by autoimmune atrophy of the adrenal, NOR with feedback ACTH hypersecretion.)

ADRENAL MEDULLA TUMORS
Pheochromocytoma and neuroblastoma. (NOT carcinoid, nor follicular adenoma.)

PHEOCHROMOCYTOMA
This occurs in the adrenal *medulla*. It presents with: increased catecholamines like epinephrine, metanephrine, normetanephrine, and vanilylmanololic acid. It will produce severe hypertension, congestive heart failure, MI, and cerebral hemorrhage. Prior to surgical correction, the patient is given Clonidine to suppress the catecholamines—if no suppression, then it is confirmed *pheochromocytoma*. Associated with MEN syndromes.

21-HYDROXYLASE DEFICIENCY
This enzyme deficiency results from a *congenital* adrenal hyperplasia (CAH). It causes *decreased* urinary 17-hydroxy*cortico*steroids, increased urinary 17-ketogenic steroids, and increased urinary 17-*ketosteroids*. (Increased androgens, and decreased glucocorticoids.) The patient may present as a young female hermaphrodite with: decreased-to-normal 17-hydroxyl corticosteroids, *increased* 17-**keto** steroids, and decreased to normal serum cortisol. There is a loss of diurnal variation. This is the most frequent cause of adrenogenital syndrome in children.

[NOTE: Cortisol deficiency seen with Congenital Adrenal Hyperplasia is associated with virilization and salt wasting—from a lack of aldosterone. It is also associated with HLA-B, and DR-1. CAH causes 11-hydroxylase deficiency and 17-hydroxylase deficiency.]

11-HYDROXYLASE DEFICIENCY
This enzyme deficiency results in an increase in *androgens* and therefore, virilization. Furthermore, hypertension and decreased potassium. The increased mineralocorticoids increase the NaCl.

17-HYDROXYLASE DEFICIENCY
This enzyme deficiency results in hypertension and a decrease in the potassium (increased mineralocorticoids). Male pseudohermaphrodism is associated with 17-hydroxylase deficiency.

THYMUS

THYMIC NEOPLASMS
90% of thymic neoplasms are *benign*. It presents with: red cell aplasia, collagen vascular diseases, Myasthenia Gravis, and chronic inflammatory disorders like Grave's disease. It is associated with: retrosternal pressure, cough, dysphagia, or simply asymptomatic. The most common *thymoma* is located in the *anterosuperior mediastinum*.

THYMOMA
A thymoma is commonly asymptomatic, and is located in the *anterior* mediastinum (chest wall "pressure sensation"). Thymoma is associated with: red cell aplasia, Myasthenia Gravis, polymyositis, and is usually *benign* (NOT malignant).

DiGEORGE'S SYNDROME
This syndrome includes: thymus agenesis with parathyroid agenesis, and immunodeficiency.

THYROID

HASHIMOTO'S THYROIDITIS
Hashimoto's Thyroiditis is associated with HLA-**DR5**, SLE, anti-microsomal antibodies, lymphoid follicles formed in the thyroid, and a variable thyroid function (it goes from **eu**thyroid to a hypothyroid state). It is more common in females than males. Hurthle cell change and interstitial fibrosis can occur. Thyroid antibody is present in the serum.

PAPILLARY THYROID CANCER
This is the most common thyroid cancer, and has the best prognosis (best 10-year survival). It is known to be induced by ionizing radiation, this was associated with "radiation to the neck as a child." It occurs more commonly in *females* than males. The metastasis is to regional lymphatics (it does NOT

secrete calcitonin). On microscopic examination, look for "**p**sammoma bodies," and "ground-glass" nuclei.

MEDULLARY CARCINOMA OF THE THYROID
This is a neuroendocrine carcinoma that is often familial, derived from **C** cells that may secrete **c**alcitonin. *Calcitonin* is the main secretory product of *medullary* carcinoma of the *thyroid*. The cancer contains amyloid stroma, and is associated with pheochromocytoma (NO psammoma bodies).

PRIMARY HYPOTHYROIDISM
Look for *decreased* T_4 and T_3 and therefore, an *increase* in TSH (to stimulate the production of more T_4). Remember, T_4 = thyroxine, and T_3 = triiodothyronine. Hypothyroid individuals have the following characteristics: *cold* intolerance, bradycardia, and obesity; increased TSH, (since no feedback inhibition of the pituitary). Both T_4 (thyroxine) and T_3 are *decreased* (25% have normal T_3), iodine uptake is decreased. It is associated with increased cholesterol; myxedema (in adults) and cretinism (in babies).

HYPERTHYROIDISM
Hyperthyroidism is caused by: diffuse thyroid hyperplasia, functioning adenoma, or excessive TSH. Antithyroid antibodies and immunologic mechanisms are important with Grave's and Hashimoto's. In the laboratory, check for an *increase* in both T_4 and T_3 with an increased RAIU (radioactive iodine uptake) and increased T_3 resin uptake. Since there is an increase in the thyroid hormones, the TSH is *decreased*. Characteristic findings in hyperthyroidism include: lid lag (the upper eyelids drag if the person quickly looks down), toxic multinodular goiter, nervousness, *heat* intolerance, increase in body temperature, atrial fibrillation, increased heart rate, and weight loss—despite an increased appetite.

GRAVE'S DISEASE
Hyperthyroidism that presents with *decreased* TSH, increased T_4, increased T_3 resin uptake, + LATS, and *decreased* cholesterol. It is most common in young women. Atrial fibrillation may occur, and *exophthalmos* may or may not be present. *Goiter* is common.

PRIMARY MYXEDEMA
This is adult hypothyroidism, with decreased total T_4, and decreased T_3 resin uptake. Therefore, we see an increased TSH. There are antithyroid antibodies present.

ENDEMIC GOITER
Caused by *decreased* iodine *intake* (NOT an error of iodine metabolism). It is an enlarged thyroid gland, but the individual is **eu**thyroid.

IODINE DEFICIENCY
This is the cause of diffuse or colloid goiter, and nodular goiter (NOT Riedel's struma, and NOT exophthalmic goiter).

Euthyroid Pregnant Woman
A **eu**thyroid pregnant woman can have: a *normal* TSH and a normal free thyroxin index (FTI), *decreased* T_3 resin uptake, and increased total serum thyroxin (T_4).

Free Thyroxin Index
The free thyroxin index is the most reliable indicator of thyroid function.

T_3 Resin Uptake Test
The T_3 resin uptake test most directly measures unoccupied sites of TBG (thyroxin binding globulin).

T_3 Suppression Test
In a normal person, this test will *decrease* the serum TSH.

PARATHYROID

*H*YPER*PARATHYROIDISM*
An increase in PTH secretion is associated with: peptic ulcer, pathologic fractures, acute pancreatitis, osteitis fibrosa cystica, renal stones (nephrocalcinosis), and hypercalcemia (NOT tetany—usually with low calcium). The most common cause is by *parathyroid adenoma*. It is part of the paraneoplastic syndrome, and is caused by APUDomas, and increased ACTH. It results in an increased serum calcium, *decreased* renal *absorption* of phosphate and *increased* phosphate *excretion*. Therefore, *decreased* serum phosphate. Also, increased cAMP and mild hyperchloremic metabolic acidosis with moderate azotemia (increased BUN and Creatinine due to a decreased GFR).

Primary Hyper*para*thyroidism
Primary hyperparathyroidism increases the PTH, and therefore, the calcium increases. Furthermore, the phophate and calcium urine excretion increases. It is associated with: *hyper*calcemia and hypercalci*u*ria, nephrocalcinosis, *hypo*phosphatemia, *increased* alkaline phosphatase activity, osteitis fibrosa cystica, and peptic ulcer (NOT tetany).

Secondary Hyper*para*thyroidism
This is hyperparathyroidism caused by: a deficiency of active Vitamin D (*decreased Vitamin D_3*), decreased serum calcium, or *increased* serum alkaline phosphatase activity. It occurs secondary to renal osteodystrophy in *chronic renal failure*—since the decreased Vitamin D results in a compensatory increase in PTH.

*H*YPO*PARATHYROIDISM*
Hypoparathyroidism is associated with: *tetany* as a result of a *decreased* serum calcium, cataracts, change in mental status, and can be caused by accidental removal of the parathyroids during thyroidectomy. It is also caused by autoimmune mechanisms, like DiGeorge Syndrome (NOT caused by chronic renal failure).

PRIMARY GOUT

Undefined enzyme defect that may be due to: increased breakdown of hematopoietic cells, increased production of *purines*, excessive dietary purine, and decreased urinary excretion of uric acid.

GLIOBLASTOMA MULTIFORME

This is the most common *glioma* in *adults*. Occurs most commonly in the *cerebrum* (NOT the cerebellum). Histologically, there are areas of necrosis with pseudopalisading.

ACROMEGALY

Acromegaly can be caused by an eosinophilic adenoma, and is due to an excess of *growth hormone* (somatotropin).

PLEOMORPHIC ADENOMA OF PAROTID GLAND

This is a benign neoplasm. Recurrence after surgical resection is mostly due to failure to resect the tumor *completely*. The parotid gland is the most common area for salivary gland tumors.

AMELOBLASTOMA

This tumor originates from odontogenic epithelium. It is more common in the *mandible* than the maxilla. Local recurrence may occur after curettage. There is peripheral palisading with myxoid center. (It does NOT produce lymph node metastases.)

DIABETES MELLITUS

*Increased pre-beta*lipoprotein in hyperlipidemia of DM. Hyalinization of islets of Langerhans. Armanni-Ebstein lesion, with a thickened basement membrane. Complications include: myocardial infarct, cerebral vascular accident (CVA), gangrene, and necrotizing papillitis. *Screen* diabetes with: Glucose in the urine, FSG, or 2-hour postprandial glucose. *Diagnose* diabetes with: Glucose Tolerance Test (GTT), and Fasting Serum Glucose (FSG). In the lab, you will find a FSG to be > 140 mg/dl, and GTT over 200 at 2 hours.

Diabetes affects many organ systems. Diabetes may lead to eventual blindness, cardiovascular diseases, renal disease, and impotence (NOT silicosis, NOT amyloidosis). Renal lesions include: necrotizing renal papillitis (papillary necrosis), arteriolosclerosis, diffuse glomerular sclerosis, *nodular glomerulosclerosis*, pyelonephritis, and glycogen deposits in the tubular cells (NOT rapidly progressive glomerulonephritis) (*see Fig. 6-1*). Lower extremity infections are caused by aerobes and anaerobes, and ischemia predisposes to these infections. In diabetes mellitus, the most common cause of death is a *myocardial infarction*.

A child born to a diabetic mother will have an increased birth weight, and an increased occurrence of hyaline membrane disease (NOT hepato/splenomegaly). Hypoglycemia in a diabetic causes tremulousness, weakness and loss of consciousness.

Juvenile Onset DM (IDDM, Type I)
Type I DM is associated with HLA haplotypes DR3 and DR4 of chromosome 6. There is an increased incidence with Hashimoto's thyroiditis, and Addison's disease; considered autoimmune disease. On lab examination, anti-islet cell antibodies may indicate a loss of pancreatic function. Furthermore, mononuclear cell infiltrates occur in the islets of Langerhans. These individuals are susceptible to developing ketoacidosis (dehydration, coma, metabolic acidosis); therefore, Type I diabetics are considered *ketosis prone*. Remember, these individuals have an absolute *lack* of insulin, and are *insulin dependent*. (They are NOT obese.)

Maturity Onset DM (NIDDM, Type II) (Fig. 6-1)
Family history (multifactorial inheritance) of diabetes is common, it is also *age* and *weight* (obesity) related. Type II diabetics may have a postreceptor defect or impaired secretion of insulin due to *decreased* number of insulin *receptors*. On lab examination, there may be renal thickening of the glomerular basement membrane. Other associated problems include: retinal microaneurysms, *amyloidosis* of the islets of Langerhans, B-cell degranulation, and they are often *Obese*. Therefore, treatment includes dietary control of body weight and if the glucose levels are not controlled, *oral hypoglycemics* may offer a solution. (Type II diabetics Do NOT usually require insulin, there is NO association with HLA haplotypes, it is NOT considered a viral or autoimmune disease, and they are NOT predisposed for ketosis.)

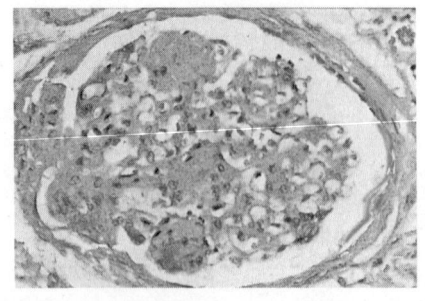

Figure 6-1. Diabetic nodular glomerulosclerosis. Kimmelstiel-Wilson nodules are present in the glomerulus. These glomerular changes result from diabetes mellitus. (For a color version see Color Plate 14.)

Nervous System   7

TABES DORSALIS

Tabes dorsalis occurs as damage to the *sensory* nerves in *dorsal* roots. This degeneration of the *posterior columns* presents with locomotor ataxia—loss of pain and joint position sense.

NEUROFIBRILLARY TANGLES

Neurofibrillary tangles are seen in: Alzheimer's disease, Down's syndrome, and normal aging (NOT in Multiple Sclerosis, NOR in Huntington's chorea).

PILOCYTIC ASTROCYTOMA

This is usually in the *cerebellum* and the floor and walls of the 3d and 4th ventricles, that affect the optic nerves. It is usually *benign* and affects children.

MENINGIOMA

This is a slow-growing tumor of the meninges (it does NOT invade the cerebral cortex). A meningioma is rare in childhood. It will cause symptoms by compression, and it is usually curable. Because of its slow growth, it may be asymptomatic until it is very large. This also increases the difficulty to remove the tumor completely and the tumor will be likely to recur. It is more common in women. On examination, it may show *psammoma bodies*.

OLIGODENDROGLIOMA

This is like a glioblastoma, that occurs in mid-life age and in the cerebral hemisphere. The presence of psammoma bodies and the invasion of the tumor and metastasis to other parts of the body may occur.

CRANIOPHARYNGIOMA

This may lead to hypopituitarism, its origin is from the Rathke's pouch, and it is frequently calcified. Its squamous epithelium and reticular stroma make it appear like tooth enamel. It occurs in children and young adults. (It is NOT usually malignant.)

GLIOBLASTOMA MULTIFORME

This is the most common glioma (primary intracranial neoplasm), and it occurs in *adults* in the *cerebrum*. This is a rapidly growing tumor.

MEDULLOBLASTOMA

This is the most common posterior fossa tumor in *children*. This *rapidly* growing tumor occurs in the *cerebellum*.

ACOUSTIC NEURINOMA

Acoustic neurinoma is similar to neurofibromatosis (it is a *bilateral* neurofibroma). This neurinoma characteristically shows: palisading and café au lait spots. (It is NOT more common in children, and does NOT contain giant cells.)

HOLOPROSENCEPHALY

This is characterized by: undivided prosencephalon, microcephaly, and harelip (NOT simian crease).

LEIGH'S SYNDROME

Subacute necrotizing encephalomyelopathy. This is an autosomal recessive syndrome of: necrosis of the *thalamus*, midbrain, pons, medulla and spine. It decreases the mitochondrial energy and patients present with weakness, seizures, and eventually death.

HUNTINGTON'S DISEASE

This is an autosomal dominant disorder that has an onset at 20 to 50 years of age. It is associated with Chromosome **4**. There is an increased calcium entry into the cell (NMDA receptors). It is associated with atrophy of the caudate nucleus. These individuals usually have a *small brain*, and have jerky, hyperkinetic choreiform movements with *dementia*.

HIV INFECTIONS

These are associated with: primary cerebral (CNS) lymphomas, cerebral candidosis, and progressive multifocal leukoencephalopathy (NOT cerebral aneurysms).

PERIVENOUS INFLAMMATORY DEMYELINATION

This demyelination may follow: measles, scarlet fever, and mumps (but, NOT rabies).

WERNICKE'S ENCEPHALOPATHY

Wernicke's encephalopathy often involves the *mammillary bodies*. It is related to *thiamine deficiency*. (Necrosis of cortex is NOT common, and it is NOT associated with posterolateral degeneration of the spinal cord.)

CONGENITAL HYDROCEPHALUS

This is seen in: Arnold-Chiari malformation (neural tube defect), Aqueduct stenosis, and Dandy-Walker syndrome (brainstem anomaly). (It is NOT seen in Marfan's syndrome.)

PURULENT MENINGITIS

Meningitis may be complicated by: chronic leptomeningitis, vasculitis, hydrocephalus, and increased intracranial pressure. Spinal fluid will show: *increased* protein, and PMNs. Therefore, *decreased* glucose.

MENINGITIS

Streptococcus pneumoniae is the most common cause of pyogenic meningitis in trauma and in the very young or old. *Klebsiella* can be the cause of meningitis in immunosuppressed patients. Remember, fulminant meningitis in a teenager (military recruit) is most likely caused by *Neisseria meningitidis*. *E. coli* is most common in neonatal meningitis. *Haemophilus influenzae* meningitis is most common in children from ages 6 months to 3 years. Meningitis can be associated with *Cryptococcus*.

SUBDURAL HEMATOMA

This hematoma results from tearing of the "bridge" veins. When an individual appears confused and inattentive, this can result from trauma, old age, and alcoholism (usually secondary to trauma). Remember, the bridging veins provide blood flow between the dura and the arachnoid.

HYPERTENSIVE CEREBRAL HEMORRHAGE

The most common location is *lenticulostriate area*, and it occurs at the *basal ganglia*.

POLIOMYELITIS

This occurs at the *anterior* horns of *spinal cord*. Poliomyelitis virus infection attacks the *lower* motor neurons. This may lead to *flaccid* paralysis, hyporeflexia, and muscle wasting.

MULTIPLE SCLEROSIS (MS)

MS is primary myelin degeneration, and has an onset at 20 to 40 years of age with *relapses*. Early on, the disease presents around small veins and venules. Usually the demyelination is periventricular, but it can occur anywhere in the brain. Multiple areas of demyelination are called *plaques*. The plaques have loss of myelin, relatively preserved axons, and astrocytic fibrosis (NOT Lewy bodies, nor argentophilic eosinophilic inclusions). MS presents as a selective degeneration of myelin, and has an increased CSF protein with oligoclonal IgG. It is more common in higher temperature locations (along the Equator), and has an increased occurrence of optic neuritis. It does have a preservation of axons in the plaque of demyelination (NOT peripheral nerve involvement).

ALZHEIMER'S DISEASE

There is association with: Chromosome 21 (related to Down's), apo E-4 gene, dementia, neurofibrillary tangles, neuritic or senile plaques, cerebral atrophy, aging, decreased Acetylcholine, and abnormal amyloid gene expression (NOT Negri bodies, nor Lewy bodies).

VON RECKLINGHAUSEN'S DISEASE

Also known as Multiple neurofibromatosis. It is associated with: an increased risk of other tumors (medullary carcinoma of the thyroid, pheochromocytomas, and intracranial neoplasms), congenital malformations, Lisch nodules (pigmented iris), malignant transformation, and "café-au-lait" spots—pigmentation over the nerve trunks. It is also associated with: decreased I.Q., skin and skeletal lesions.

PARKINSON'S DISEASE

This presents as a degeneration of the *dopaminergic* neurons of the *substantia nigra*. Therefore, a reduced Dopamine is corrected with L-DOPA treatment. Microscopically, *Lewy bodies* are seen (Figs. 7-1 and 7-2). Also, look for a "pill-rolling" tremor and irregular gait. It has been associated with MPTP, a street drug (toxin) that affects the nigrostriatal-dopaminergic system.

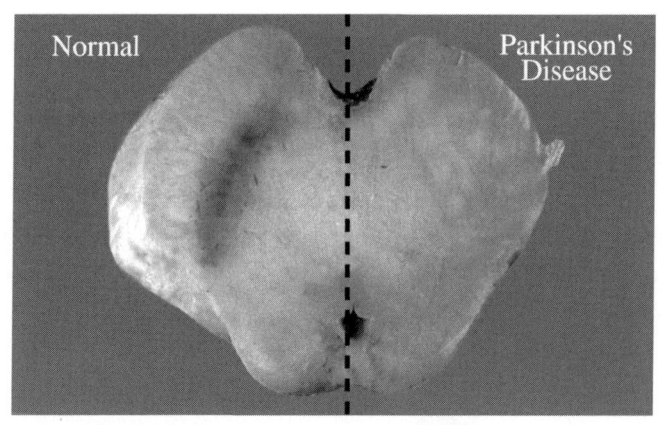

Figure 7-1. Normal versus Parkinson's Disease. In Parkinson's disease, there is a degeneration of pigmented nerve cells in the substantia nigra. Normal pigmented substantia nigra at the midbrain level. (This figure compares one side each of a normal and a Parkinson's-affected brain. In the actual slice, the sides would be mirror images.) (For a color version see Color Plate 15.)

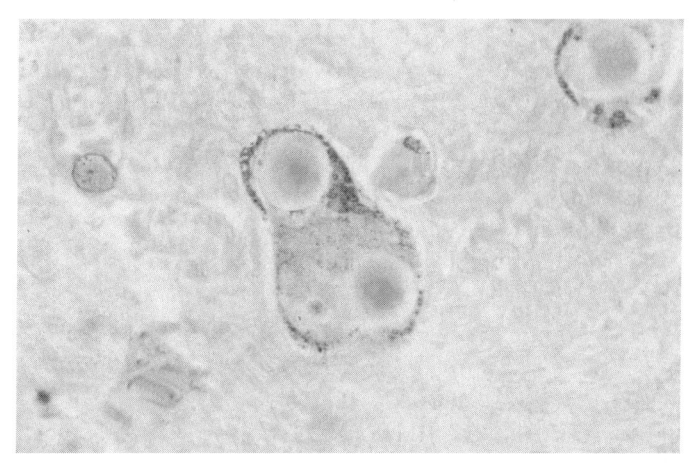

Figure 7-2. Parkinson's Disease. Idiopathic destruction of neurons in the substantia nigra. Lewy body (*center*): this pink-staining inclusion is found in the neurons of the substantia nigra from a patient with Parkinson's disease. (For a color version see Color Plate 16.)

Genitourinary   8

GLOMERULAR AND TUBULAR DISEASES

NEPHRITIC SYNDROME
Nephritic syndrome presents as: hematuria (with red cell casts), mild proteinuria, hypertension and increased wbc's in the urine. It is typified by post-streptococcal (proliferative) glomerulonephritis, and most patients recover completely. Remember, antibodies to *streptococcus* antigens will form immune complexes and localize in the kidney (*immune complex deposition*).

ACUTE PROLIFERATIVE GLOMERULONEPHRITIS
This acute nephritic syndrome occurs approximately 1–2 weeks after a strep infection of the throat or skin. This GMN presents as: swollen, hypercellular glomeruli, with azotemia and hematuria (increased rbc casts in urine). There is an increased anti-streptococcal exoenzyme titer (increased ASO titer). 95% of the children recover. Look for the "starry sky" pattern or "humplike" IgA immunoglobulin deposits at the **sub**epithelial side of the glomerular *basement membrane* (NO linear immunofluorescence).

MEMBRANOPROLIFERATIVE GLOMERULONEPHRITIS
This occurs as *thickened* capillary loops and *proliferation* of the glomerular cells. Type I presents as a mix of nephritic and nephrotic syndromes, with sub**endo**thelial and sub**epi**thelial, and mesangial deposits of C3. Type II presents as ribbon-like electron-dense material with sub**epi**thelial deposits.

FOCAL GLOMERULONEPHRITIS
This is *focal* to only some of the *glomeruli* that are damaged and proliferative.

CHRONIC GLOMERULONEPHRITIS
This is the "end-stage" glomerular disease that occurs from post-streptococcal GMN, membranous GMN and others. It is the most common cause of *chronic renal failure*.

INTERSTITIAL NEPHRITIS
This occurs from the use of drugs like: *phenacetin with other analgesics*, ampicillin, furosemide, and various other drugs. Remember, analgesic abuse nephritis. Clinically, the patient may present with: fever, rash, azotemia, pyuria, and hematuria. Phenacetin mixtures (phenacetin, aspirin, and/or acetaminophen) may cause papillary necrosis and tubulointerstitial nephritis.

HEREDITARY NEPHRITIS
An example is Alport's Syndrome, which includes: GMN with nerve deafness, lens dislocation, cataracts, and corneal dystrophy.

NEPHROTIC SYNDROME
Nephrotic syndrome presents as: excessive permeability of glomerular capillary wall to proteins—proteinuria or increased protein excretion (> 3.5 g/day), hypoalbuminemia, and edema without azotemia. It is caused by: membranous glomerulonephritis (GMN) or IgA nephropathy, lipoid nephrosis, focal segmental glomerulosclerosis, SLE, amyloidosis, and drugs like gold and penicillamine.

LIPOID NEPHROSIS
Also known as *minimal change disease*. This is the most common cause of nephrotic syndrome of children. It occurs after a respiratory infection, and is associated with proteinuria and *lipid* droplets in the tubules (leading to lipid in the urine). Lipoid nephrosis has normal glomeruli, but diffuse foot processes of the visceral epithelial cells (NO immunoglobulin deposits). These patients have an excellent to good long-term prognosis, and have a dramatic response to corticosteroid therapy.

BERGER'S DISEASE
Also known as IgA Nephropathy. It is characterized by deposits of IgA in the mesangial region (mesangial proliferation). Initially, there is benign recurrent hematuria. This eventually leads to *chronic* renal failure over the next couple of decades. Berger's disease presents with: deposits of Ig**A** in the mesangium and benign hematuria.

FOCAL SEGMENTAL GLOMERULOSCLEROSIS
This is the cause of nephrosis (proteinuria), and therefore, sclerosis of *some* of the glomeruli (focal). It presents with IgM and C3 deposition.

IMMUNE COMPLEX DEPOSITS SEEN WITH:
Membranous glomerulonephritis, and diffuse proliferative form of lupus nephropathy. (NOT with lipoid nephrosis)

INCREASED WIDTH OF GLOMERULAR BASEMENT MEMBRANE
Diabetes mellitus, and membranous glomerulonephritis. (NOT acute poststreptococcus glomerulonephritis, NOT Berger's disease.)

SLE (SYSTEMIC LUPUS ERYTHEMATOSUS)
In SLE, look for concentric rings of collagen around splenic arterioles, "wireloop" lesions of glomerular capillaries. It is associated with atypical nonbac-

terial verucous endocarditis (NOT esophageal stenosis—as is seen in scleroderma). Lupus nephropathy shows **subendo**thelial immune complex deposition and the "wire loops" (Fig. 8-1).

SLE can present with: lymphadenopathy, a *false positive* serologic test for *Syphilis*, nephrotic syndrome, non-bacterial (atypical verrucous) endocarditis. Usually, the patient is a young female. Look for hematoxylin bodies, and fibrinoid deposits in the blood vessels, and with focal glomerulonephritis. A drug-induced SLE-like syndrome can occur with: hydralazine, procainamide, isoniazid, and D-penicillamine.

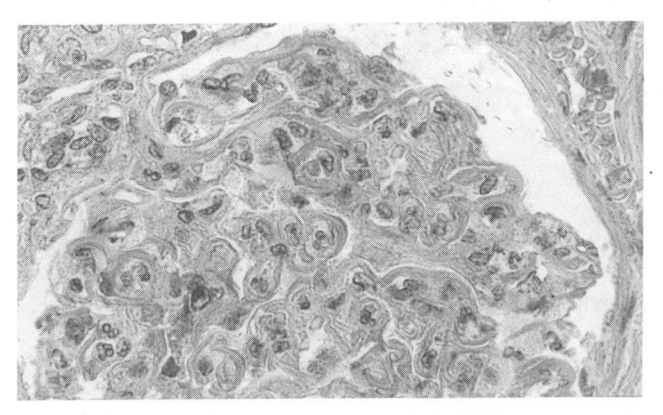

Figure 8-1 SLE and Lupus Nephropathy. Subendothelial immune complex deposition and thickening of the glomerular basement membrane—"wire-loop" lesions. (For a color version see Color Plate 17.)

RENAL INSUFFICIENCY

Renal disease in the earliest stages, near renal failure. Use tests that detect: serum creatinine concentration, creatinine clearance, urine osmolality following a fluid fast. (NOT serum uric acid concentration)

ACUTE RENAL FAILURE

During acute renal failure, look for suppressed renal function, *oliguria*, and decreased blood pressure. (The first sign is losing the concentrating ability of urine.) Renal failure is often caused by acute tubular necrosis (neprotoxicosis from drugs) which causes ischemia and shock. Acute renal failure is therefore a result of this hypotension and is *reversible*. Renal failure may occur with multiple myeloma.

RENAL TUBULOINTERSTITIAL LESIONS

These lesions are associated with: hyperparathyroidism, multiple myeloma, hypervitaminosis D, and analgesic abuse.

RENAL PAPILLARY NECROSIS

This is associated with: diabetes mellitus and may cause transient obstructive uropathy. (It does NOT occur from renal artery stenosis, and is NOT associated with RBC casts in the urine.)

ACUTE TUBULAR NECROSIS

Acute tubular necrosis appears as acute renal failure with oliguria. Look for granular casts, oliguria, a possible mismatched blood transfusion, DIC, or crush injuries. In the lab, check for: azotemia, oliguria, and a FE (Fractional excretion) of sodium > 20 % (NOT anemia).

AZOTEMIA

This is an increase in serum concentrations of creatinine and urea (increased BUN). Therefore, you will find increased *nitrogenous waste* products in the blood. Prerenal azotemia has a decrease in effective blood volume, and congestive heart failure. For example, acute renal failure will cause azotemia with oliguria or anuria.

UREMIA

Uremia is azotemia with clinical signs and symptoms that appear like chronic renal failure. The stage of renal disease is indicated by: creatinine clearance, fibrinous pericarditis, metabolic acidosis, decreased serum calcium levels, GI inflammation (gastritis), ulceration, and bleeding.

HYPERURICEMIA

This is caused by thiazides, furosemide (diuretic) treatment, polycythemia vera, and Lesch-Nyhan Syndrome (hereditary hyperuricemia). Hyperuricemia appears from the overproduction of uric acid, decreased renal excretion of uric acid, hemolytic anemia, and leukemia.

RENIN

Angiotensinogen is activated to Angiotensin I by renin. The renin release is increased with hypovolemia or low blood pressure. Angiotensin I (AI) is converted by *angiotensin converting enzyme (ACE)* to Angiotensin II which is a stimulator of *aldosterone* secretion. Aldosterone then increases the NaCl reabsorption and potassium excretion (increased serum NaCl and decreased potassium). (Therefore, renin is NOT a precursor of AII, and is NOT stimulated by aldosterone release.)

BASEMENT MEMBRANE THICKENING

Thickening of the basement membrane occurs in diffuse diabetic glomerular sclerosis, membranous nephritis, and SLE (NOT in minimal change lipoid nephrosis).

CHILDHOOD HEMOLYTIC UREMIC SYNDROME

This causes acute renal failure in children, a flu-like syndrome, with thrombi in the glomerular capillaries.

RENAL INFARCT

An occlusion of the artery in the kidney will cause a *wedge-shaped* infarct. The area that the artery normally supplies then becomes pale, and the border will become hyperemic. Eventually, the affected area is replaced with scar tissue. Renal infarcts are caused by *emboli* that obstruct the artery (Fig. 8-2).

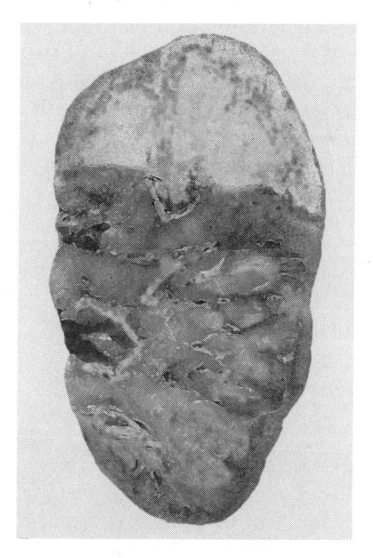

Figure 8-2 Renal Infarct. Area of infarction from arterial vascular occlusion and ischemia (*pale area*); usually appearing as a wedge-shaped area. Hyperemic area develops around the area of infarction, then after 10 days granulation tissue forms and scarring develops. Normal, unaffected portion of kidney (*lower third*). (For a color version see Color Plate 18.)

RENAL STONES

RENAL CALCULI
Renal calculi are usually calcium-phosphate-oxalate stones, and are formed by: increased cystine excretion, hyperparathyroidism—increased calcium, and

gout—increased uric acid (NOT by hemolytic anemia). The triple-struvite stones are composed of: magnesium-ammonium-phosphate. These are considered "Staghorn stones". These Staghorn (struvite) stones conform to the outline of the renal calyces. Others include: uric acid stones and cystine stones.

ACUTE CHOLECYSTITIS
Consider this inflammation of the *gall bladder* in any obese, 30–60 y/o female, who presents with right upper quadrant (RUQ) pain, and the gallbladder is palpable (enlarged). The gallstones may obstruct the neck of the gall bladder, and may even cause perforation.

CYSTIC DISEASES

POLYCYSTIC RENAL DISEASE (ADULT TYPE)
This is an autosomal *dominant* disease (positive family history) that is associated with: many *bi*lateral cysts in liver (it involves *both* kidneys, and is NOT unilateral), massively enlarged kidneys, renal failure, berry aneurysms, and hypertension (Fig. 8-3). It progresses to renal insufficiency in the *middle age*. It is more common than infantile polycystic renal disease. Consider this disease in a patient who may present as a 50 year old with *palpable kidneys*, renal *infection*, and *hypertension*. Death may be due to renal failure, hypertension, a subarachnoid hemorrhage, or a rupture of a cerebral aneurysm.

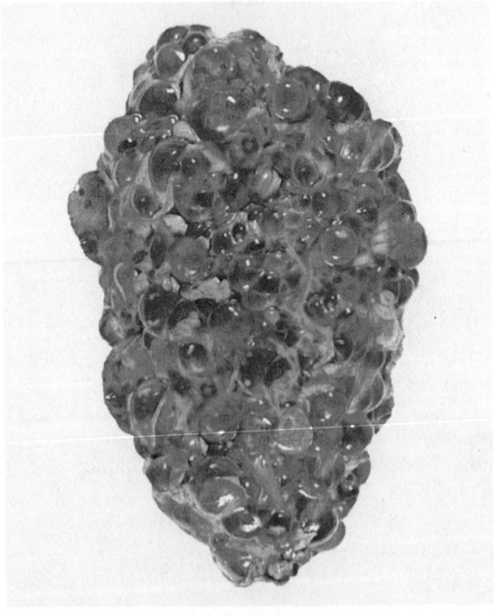

Figure 8-3 Adult Polycystic Renal Disease. Enlarged cystic kidneys (only one shown) resulting in renal failure, pain, and hypertension. The kidneys develop polycystic changes (filled with cysts) that may hemorrhage and create hematuria and progressive renal failure. (For a color version see Color Plate 19.)

Polycystic Renal Disease (Infantile Type)

This is an autosomal *recessive* disease that is seen in infants (< 2 years old) and has a poor prognosis because of its rapid renal failure in childhood. The kidneys are enlarged and cystic, and the liver may also have cysts. It is associated with neonatal respiratory distress syndrome (hyaline membrane disease). (It is NOT X-linked recessive, and is NOT caused by extrarenal urinary obstruction).

INFECTIONS

Urinary Tract Infection (UTI)

UTI's are considered either an infection of the *bladder* which is considered *cystitis*, or an infection of the *kidneys* which is considered *pyelonephritis*. *Upper* urinary tract infections usually occur as *multiple* infections, and in females. Factors include: functionally inadequate urogenital secretory immunoglobulins, and mucosal receptors for enterobacteria (NOT from excessive sexual intercourse).

Acute Pyelonephritis

This is an acute urinary tract infection (an infection of the kidney). There will be many *white cell casts* present in the *urine specimen*. White blood cells are in clumps and casts, and bacteria are found in the fresh specimen. Also, there is a decreased concentrating ability. Eventually this may lead to *chronic pyelonephritis*, where inflammation will cause scars to the kidney and *tubular necrosis* from repeated inflammation.

TRANSITIONAL CELL CARCINOMA OF THE BLADDER

With transitional cell carcinoma, consider *occupational exposure* to environmental agents (the carcinogen is excreted in the urine) which include: cigarettes, *aniline dyes*, and rubber products (tire manufacturing). Transitional cell carcinoma may also be seen in the urethra, ureter, and renal pelvis.

RENAL CELL CARCINOMA

Consider renal cell carcinoma in a patient with: *hematuria*, polycythemia, costovertebral pain, and fever. It often invades the renal veins. (Usually, it does NOT occur in children.)

DESMOPLASIA

This is the overproduction of fibroblasts and fibrous connective tissue. It may be seen as tumor induction of fibrous stroma.

EXFOLIATIVE CYTOLOGY

Procedure most important for observed decreased prevalence of invasive carcinoma of uterine cervix.

URINARY BLADDER TUMORS

These are characteristically *transitional* cell carcinomas. They are aggressive tumors that lack blood group antigens on the surface of tumor cells. *Cyclophosphamide*, tobacco, *azo* dyes, and analgesics have been known to be related to carcinoma of the bladder (usually papillary *transitional* cell carcinoma). *Squamous* cell carcinoma may be seen with an infection by *Schistosoma haematobium* of the bladder. β-Glucoronidase in the bladder mucosa may convert some carcinogens to *active* carcinogens.

WILM'S TUMOR OF THE KIDNEY

Wilm's tumor is most common in *children* 2–4 years old. This tumor of the urinary system has the clinical sign of nephrotic syndrome. The first sign is usually a *large* palpable abdominal mass. It presents with abdominal pain, hematuria, and a palpable mass. You may see other congenital anomalies, like aniridia (missing iris) and hemihypertrophy. This has been associated with *deletions* of the *short* arm of chromosome **11**. Wilm's tumor of the kidney has many cell and tissue components originating from *mesoderm*. It has primitive glomeruli (renal tubules) and abortive tubules, within a spindle cell stroma. This is an aggressive tumor, but with proper surgery and radiation/chemotherapy, it has a good cure rate—very good long-term survival after treatment.

REPRODUCTIVE

OVARIES
Most common site of endometriosis externa.

OVARIAN TUMORS THAT PRODUCE ENDOCRINE EFFECTS:
Granulosa cell tumor, Sertoli-Leydig cell tumor, struma ovarii, and choriocarcinoma.

SEX CORD-STROMAL TUMORS

Sertoli-Leydig cell tumor
Ovarian neoplasms that cause amenorrhea and hirsutism. Usually, this occurs **uni**laterally, and acts like testes cells (giving male-like symptoms).

Granulosa cell tumor
This is an estrogen-producing ovarian tumor (giving female-like symptoms). It may present in a female child with precocious puberty, a 10-cm firm, smooth, right ovarian mass palpable on a pelvic exam. Or in a 60 year old (post-menopausal) female with *irregular* uterine bleeding, and a *palpable* ovarian mass. Usually, it occurs in a post-menopausal female as a solid, unilateral tumor—all of these tumors are potentially malignant. They are predisposed to *endometrial carcinoma*.

Meig's Syndrome
Look for the triad of: ovarian tumor, ascites, and hydrothorax. This unilateral *fibroma* (tumor) is usually a solid grayish-white mass.

TESTICULAR TUMORS
Choriocarcinoma associated with gynecomastia. The majority are *germ cell tumors*, and the remaining are sex cord–stromal tumors.

Seminoma
This is a testicular tumor that produces gonadotropins (i.e., hCG or human chorionic gonadotropin).

Choriocarcinoma
This is also a testicular tumor that produces gonadotropins. Choriocarcinoma may follow a hydatiform form mole or a normal ectopic pregnancy. It is characterized by early widespread metastasis, and is associated with Thecal-lutein cysts. It is a highly malignant tumor.

CRYPTORCHIDISM
This often presents as a unilateral problem and may be a cause of *infertility*. This may become a malignancy. The patient may not even be aware of the problem. Surgical placement of testis in the scrotum does **NOT** eliminate the risk of malignancy.

PROSTATIC SPECIFIC ANTIGEN (PSA)
PSA is helpful to identify a *prostatic* origin of metastatic disease. It is principally used to monitor the therapeutic response of patients with an established diagnosis of *carcinoma of prostate*. (It is NOT useful to distinguish benign prostatic hyperplasia (BPH) from carcinoma of the prostate.)

BPH (BENIGN PROSTATIC HYPERTROPHY)
BPH occurs mostly in the *peripheral* zone *posterior* lobe. This is why you can usually palpate the prostatic hypertrophy on a rectal exam. BPH is also known as *nodular* hyperplasia. The hyperplasia occurs from gland proliferation. The periurethral inner area has an enlarged gland with *nodular* urinary tract *obstruction*. Therefore, the individual complains of frequent urine UTIs. It has an increased incidence with age.

CHRONIC PROSTATITIS
This is seen in a young patient (35 y/o) who complains of lower abdominal pain, nocturia, frequency and dysuria. On examination, his rectal exam shows an *enlarged prostate*, and culture secretions are negative. The abacterial form is the most common prostatitis. Recurrent UTI's are possibly bacterial. A pathogen that *may be* involved is *Ureaplasma urealyticum*.

CARCINOMA OF PROSTATE
This is the most common carcinoma in men. It most commonly occurs in the *peripheral* zone *posteriorly*. Therefore, it can be palpated. Lymphatic metas-

tasis may occur to the *obturator nodes*. Hematogenous spread may occur to the *bone*. Carcinoma of the prostate is associated with: trabeculation of the urinary bladder, lower back pain, *increased* BUN, serum alkaline phosphatase, and prostatic acid phosphatase. You can assess metastasis by: induction of osteoblastic activity in bone, and production of acid phosphatase. (NOT by hyperparathyroidism with lytic bone lesions, NOT by increased hCG.)

DYSGERMINOMA
This is an ovarian "testicular seminoma" that presents as a solid, unilateral, and often malignant tumor. Dysgerminoma has a *good* prognosis when it is treated.

NECROTIZING CERVICITIS
This may appear when herpetic giant cells are seen in a Pap smear with a pregnant women.

CARCINOMA OF CERVIX
Usually this is a *squamous cell carcinoma* (NOT adenocarcinoma) of the cervix. Carcinoma of the cervix has an *increased* incidence with: women with multiple sex partners (sexual intercourse transmission), HSV-2 viral herpes, Human papillomavirus type 16 and 18, early age of first intercourse, low socioeconomic standard, multiparous female, and smokers. As you can see, this is uncommon in celibate women. It usually arises at the squamocolumnar junction of the external cervical os. Dysplasia is the precursor lesion. Because of the slow development of in situ cancer (it occurs over many years), changes can be detected even before the lesion is cancer. As such, there is a dramatic decrease in the death rate due to the *Pap*anicolaou screening test. Mortality is related to local spread. Severe dysplasia of cervix should be treated aggressively.

ENDOMETRIAL ADENOCARCINOMA
Usually the patient presents with *abnormal bleeding*, and is 55–65 years old. It is associated with: estrogen-secreting ovarian tumors, hypertension, diabetes mellitus, infertility, and obesity.

OVARY
Most ovarian tumors originate from the *surface epithelium*. The ovary is the most common site of *endometriosis*.

ENDOMETRIOSIS
This occurs as endometrial glands outside of the uterus. It is associated with pelvic pain, dysmenorrhea, and infertility.

STEIN-LEVANTHAL SYNDROME
Also known as Polycystic Ovarian Syndrome. It presents as: infertility, amenorrhea, hirsutism, obesity, oligomenorrhea, anovulation (infertility), with **bi**laterally enlarged *polycystic ovaries*. This is an important cause of infertility to remember. It shows as increased androgens with cystic ovaries. Patients benefit from wedge resection. (NOT menometrorrhagia, and it does NOT follow multiple pregnancies.)

DYSFUNCTIONAL UTERINE BLEEDING
Problems with menses is seen with: endocrine disorders (like a pituitary tumor or thyroid problem), ovarian tumor (polycystic), and metabolic problems (like obesity or malnourishment).

ECTOPIC PREGNANCY
This is the most common cause of *hematosalpinx*.

UTERINE CHORIOCARCINOMA
This may be preceded by hydatidiform mole. It can arise in the testes. It may follow a normal or an ectopic pregnancy. Uterine choriocarcinoma occurs in the Far East more than in the United States. It is made of 2 cell types. Look for increased chorionic gonadotropin (hCG). This is a highly malignant carcinoma.

LEIOMYOMA
Leiomyoma is a *benign* mass of smooth muscle cells (Fig. 8-4). It is seen in a young female with *irregular*, profuse uterine bleeding and an irregularly enlarged uterus. It is least likely to become malignant nor invasive (considered benign), and is common in the uterus and GI tract (NOT common in deep soft tissues). Leiomyoma is the most common neoplasm of the *uterus*.

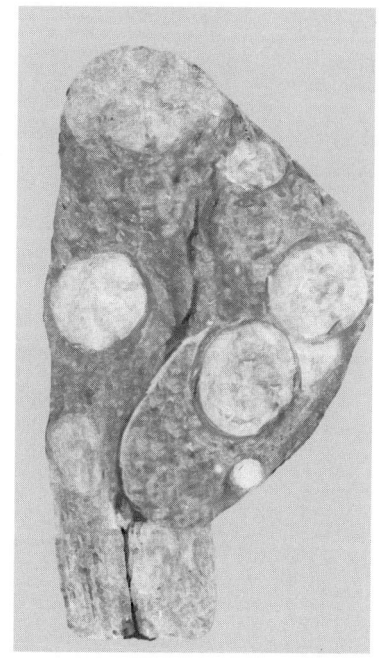

Figure 8-4 Fibroids or Leiomyomas of the Uterus. Leiomyomas are round, rubbery nodules of benign masses of smooth muscle cells. They are the most common tumors in women. Usually present in women over 30, and may be asymptomatic or with irregular, painful bleeding. (For a color version see Color Plate 20.)

Placenta Previa
This is the attachment of the *placenta lower in the uterus* than normal. Therefore, it covers the uterine os.

Abruptio Placenta
This is the premature *separation* (detachment) of the placenta.

DES (Diethylstilbestrol)
Girls whose mothers were treated with DES while pregnant will show increased occurrence of: vaginal adenosis, *clear cell adeno*carcinoma of the *vagina*. (NOT uterine leiomyoma, nor ovarian tumors)

Skin/Breast   9

SKIN

JUNCTIONAL NEVUS
A junctional nevus occurs as a small, flat brown to black skin lesion. On microscopic examination, there are spindle-shaped nevus cells at the *border* of the epidermis and dermis.

COMPOUND NEVUS
The *dermis* contains the junctional activity of melanocytes and mature nevus cells.

MELANIN
Increased melanin occurs in the skin of patients with: adrenal cortical hypofunction, hemochromatosis, and during pregnancy (NOT vitiligo—which has a decrease). The decrease in cortisol will increase the ACTH from the anterior pituitary.

LENTIGO
Lentigo occurs as benign, hyperpigmented macules (like freckles, but they do NOT darken with exposure to the sun).

PEMPHIGUS
Chronic bullous skin diseases (with *blisters* as the primary feature). It is considered an autoimmune disease. Pemphigus *vulgaris* can be fatal if left untreated. IgG antibodies occur to the intracellular cement substance of the skin (at the intercellular sites of the stratified squamous epithelium). The blisters will rupture and leave an erosion.

MOLE WITH NEVUS CELLS
When confined to the *dermis*, a mole remains *benign* throughout.

BASAL CELL CARCINOMA
Basal cell carcinoma occurs to the *sun-exposed skin*. If left untreated, this will slowly grow (gradual *local* enlargement—but, NO metastasis), and ulcerate.

Consider basal cell carcinoma in a 70-year old patient with a *locally* destructive skin lesion of the face above the ear and mouth.

PSORIASIS

Psoriasis consists of well demarcated, erythematous plaques with loose scales (lesions) (Fig. 9-1). Changes are Munro's microabcesses and parakeratosis. They may cause erythroderma (total body erythema and scales). Psoriasis is associated with elderly individuals, HLA, AIDS, and psoriasis may occur initially following trauma to the area.

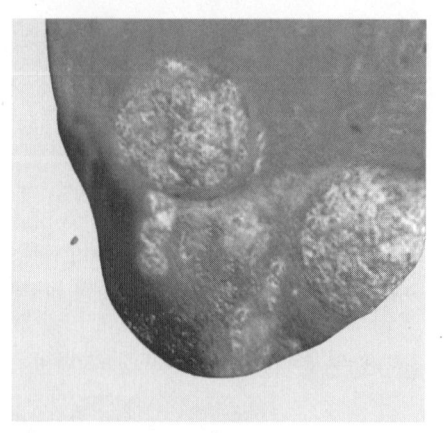

Figure 9-1 Psoriasis. Common elbow appearance of raised silver-white scales with red patching seen in this chronic skin disease. (For a color version see Color Plate 21.)

SQUAMOUS CELL CARCINOMA

This is the most common tumor of *sun-exposed skin* of the *elderly*.

Bowen's disease

This is a squamous cell carcinoma that may appear de novo or secondary to actinic keratosis. The epidermal layer has increased atypical keratinocytes, and erythematous plaques—possibly with scaling. This disease does NOT metastasize, but does require treatment by excision.

Scar carcinoma

This occurs in a past scar that suddenly has a change—like an ulceration or nodular growth.

Verrucous carcinoma

This is usually found on the plantar side of the foot. It is NOT a wart, but appears like one.

MALIGNANT MELANOMA (Fig. 9-2)

Malignant melanoma grows initially horizontally and then vertically. The extent of *vertical* growth is of concern with nodular raising. Increased incidence in fair skinned persons. The patient may notice the lesion because of a change of a pre-existing pigmented lesion. It may occur in the eye, leptomeninges, or mucosal surfaces. Lentigo maligna melanoma is a laterally spreading, irregularly pigmented lesion on the cheek of an elderly person. Treatment of malignant melanoma is by surgical excision.

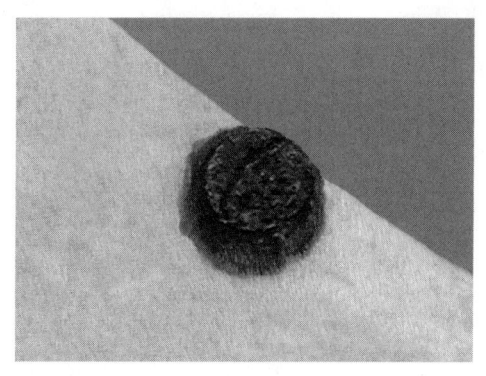

Figure 9-2 Malignant Melanoma. Large, irregular pigmented skin lesion. Notice the irregular symmetry, borders, and pigmentation. Increased risk in lightly pigmented individuals, and depth of vertical growth increases probability of metastasis. (For a color version see Color Plate 22.)

XERODERMA PIGMENTOSUM
Xeroderma pigmentosum is a rare condition that occurs as a defect in an enzyme responsible for DNA repair. This leads to misrepair of DNA and malignancy.

SQUAMOUS PAPILLOMAS
Benign neoplasms of the skin. Also considered as "skin tags."

BREAST

FIBROCYSTIC DISEASE OF THE BREAST
This is the most common breast lesion in women. It is usually **bi**lateral and is a *palpable* mass or *lumpy masses* in the breast and increased midcycle tenderness. (It is NOT greater in older age, NOT premalignant, and does NOT have encapsulated nodules.)

BREAST MASS/TUMOR
Most common location of a breast mass or tumor is the *upper-lateral (outer) quadrant*.

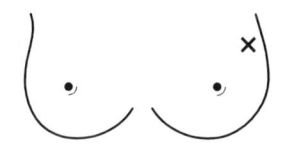

Lymph node invasion from *outer* quadrant tumors metastasize to *axillary nodes*. Tumors from the inner or center of the breast tend to metastasize to the *internal mammary nodes*. Risk factors for carcinoma of the breast include: #1 is the family history of cancer; then, age (over 40 years old), obesity (increased estrogen), **nulli**parity, alcoholism, HER-2/neu proto-oncogene, *early* menarche/late menopause, and *previous* colon, endometrial, or ovarian *cancer*. Carcinoma of the breast is the most common cancer in women. Factors of worsening prognosis of breast cancer include: increased tumor size, increased number of positive nodes for cancer, histologic type of cancer. Remember, breast cancers with *positive* estrogen *receptors* are better for therapy response— Tamoxifen has anti-estrogen effects. Cancers that are negative for estrogen receptors have higher proliferation, and do NOT respond well to these antagonists.

BENIGN BREAST LESIONS

Fibroadenoma of the breast
This is the most common breast *tumor* in females. It is a *benign* and well-demarcated mass. It is found in a *young* female (it occurs in the reproductive years) with a *freely movable, rubbery firm mass* in one breast (**uni**lateral). The size ranges from 1 to 10 cm, and it must be excised to confirm that it is a benign tumor.

Phyllodes tumor
This is a *bulky*, usually *benign* breast tumor. (Cystosarcoma phyllodes is considered a malignant tumor.)

Intraductal papilloma
This *benign* lesion usually occurs in women near *menopause*. It appears as small "raspberry-like" masses near the *nipple*, and as serous or *bloody discharge*. Also, consider intraductal papilloma in a 45-year old female with no palpable breast mass, who has *bleeding from the nipple*. Intraductal papilloma is only a few millimeters in size. There is only a risk if the individual took oral contraceptives in the past and had higher estrogen-progestin levels then was necessary—therefore, it is found in mostly in middle-aged women. A nipple adenoma occurs as fibrosis of the duct with hyperplasia. It is considered a benign lesion, but has an increased risk of developing *invasive carcinoma*. Consider *adenoma of the nipple* in a patient with a breast mass, and serous or *bloody discharge* from the nipple (it is considered a *benign* lesion).

Nipple eczematoid lesion
A patient may have an eczematoid lesion of the nipple as the sequela of radiation therapy.

CARCINOMA OF THE BREAST

Ductal carcinoma

INFILTRATING DUCTAL CARCINOMA
Also known as *invasive* ductal carcinoma. This is the most common breast *cancer* in females. It may be seen in an *older* patient (60 y/o) as

a 3-cm irregular, *fibrous* lesion. It is associated with cords of firm, grayish-white tissue that are irregular throughout adipose tissue.

INTRADUCTAL CARCINOMA
This is carcinoma of the *duct system*. The ducts appear thickened, and the *in situ* carcinoma may go through the duct wall and become invasive.

MEDULLARY CARCINOMA
This is a well-circumscribed lesion with large, *pleomorphic cells*. It is less aggressive than infiltrating carcinoma.

PAPILLARY CARCINOMA
This is a rare breast carcinoma that appears as a *lump* and may have *bloody discharge* from the nipple (like a benign papilloma).

Lobular carcinoma

LOBULAR CARCINOMA IN SITU
This is considered a **bi**lateral breast lesion that occurs in younger women before menopause. This may lead to *invasive lobular breast carcinoma*. It contains clusters of neoplastic cells that organize into the intralobular ductules and the acini. It is confined to the lobules and does NOT metastasize (but, it may develop into an invasive carcinoma).

INFILTRATING LOBULAR CARCINOMA
This is found in older patients and is seen with small cells of a linear arrangement, known as *"Indian file"* (Fig. 9-3).

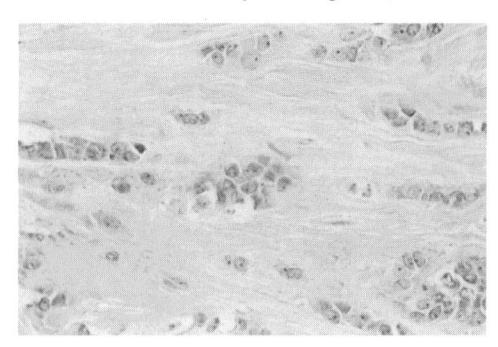

Figure 9-3 Invasive Lobular Breast Carcinoma. This breast carcinoma is usually bilateral, and histologically presents with small tumor cells in an "Indian file." (For a color version see Color Plate 23.)

Paget's disease of the breast
Eczematous skin around the nipple of older women. Most patients also have invasive carcinoma or a form of ductal carcinoma that involves the skin of the nipple or areola. Paget's disease of the nipple predicts the development of *intraductal carcinoma*.

Sarcoma

CYSTOSARCOMA PHYLLODES (MALIGNANT)
This is a *locally aggressive* tumor that may metastasize through blood vessels (blood stream). Therefore, it is NOT necessary to surgically resect axillary lymph nodes—only the mass itself.

ANGIOSARCOMA
This is another aggressive tumor that is common in younger (20–30 year olds) patients. It consists of a *bulky* breast tumor that is highly *vascular*. It has a very poor prognosis.

Inflammatory carcinoma of the breast
Inflammatory carcinoma of the breast occurs as a massive involvement of the lymphatics, with swelling and reddening ("orange skin") of the skin of the breast. There is local invasion, nipple retraction, and dimpling of the skin—with the appearance of an orange peel (this is the reason it is called *peau d' orange*).

Musculoskeletal 10

AMYOTROPHIC LATERAL SCLEROSIS (ALS)

Also known as Lou Gehrig's Disease. This is a muscle *denervation* disorder and therefore you will see *muscle atrophy*. On muscle biopsy, there are: target fibers, angulated atrophy of muscle fibers, collateral sprouting of nerves, and fiber type grouping with specific atrophy.

MYELOFIBROSIS

If it is an older patient with mild anemia and splenomegaly, check the peripheral blood smear: very decreased numbers of blast cells, decreased number of metamyelocytes, with scattered *nucleated* RBCs, and *tear-drop* shaped erythrocytes. With bone aspiration we will see: megakaryocytic hyperplasia and *fibrotic* replacement of marrow elements [but, NOT erythroid hyperplasia, and NOT myeloid (granulocytic) hyperplasia].

OSTEOSARCOMA

Most common primary tumor of the bone. Greatest growth at *epi*physeal region (at the *meta*physeal ends of the long bones—before the epiphyseal closure). Retinoblastoma is often associated with an osteosarcoma. An osteosarcoma may complicate Paget's disease. Usually the patient is a young male. Osteosarcoma is common around the *knee* joint. Metastasis usually first occurs to the *lung*.

CHONDROSARCOMA

Chondrosarcoma may be seen in a young patient with a palpable mass, and a radiolucent X-Ray that shows an osseous lesion with scalloped edges—origin near the anterior superior iliac spine. Usually the patient is greater than 35 years old since it is a slower growing tumor. It usually affects the central skeleton and the knee (NOT the ankles, nor the wrists). The chondrosarcoma may become an osteochondroma. (There are NO multinucleated giant cells, and it does NOT follow Paget's disease of the bone.)

SOLITARY OSTEOCHONDROMA

This is a *benign*, hereditary developmental anomaly that is usually seen in young patients. It usually arises in the epiphysis area.

Collagen Type	Found In:
Type I collagen	Tendon, fascia, dermis (skin), and bone.
Type II collagen	Cartilage.
Type III collagen	Reticulin, skin, embryonic dermis, and blood vessels.
Type IV collagen	The basement lamina of epithelial and endothelial cells.

SERUM ALKALINE PHOSPHATASE

Serum *alkaline* phosphatase is *increased* in: *bone* disease (like Rickets), breast carcinoma metastatic to *bone*, Paget's disease of bone, primary hyperparathyroidism, biliary obstruction (liver disease), and pregnancy (NOT with muscle wasting).

EWING'S SARCOMA

Usually seen in *young* patients (NOT in the elderly). Ewing's sarcoma resembles lymphoma histologically. It usually arises in the *midshaft* of the bone and the pelvis as it expands the cortex. A destructive periosteal *onion skinning* can occur. It originates from neuroectodermal differentiation. (It is NOT common in African-Americans, and does NOT originate from the periosteum.)

REITER'S SYNDROME

This syndrome includes a triad of: arthritis, conjunctivitis, and urethritis. It is also associated with HLA B-27, and is seen in young *males* as a cause of arthritis.

SEQUESTRUM

This is a portion of necrotic bone tissue separated from a healthy bone tissue. This is usually an area of osseous infarction.

INVOLUCRUM

This is an wrapping membrane or sheath of new bone *around* the sequestrum. It is a result of reactive new bone formation in osteomyelitis.

HYPOVITAMINOSIS D

This presents as decreased osteo*clastic* and osteo*blastic* activity, with an increased circulating PTH. (NOT radiolucent bones)

DEGENERATIVE JOINT DISEASE (DJD)

Decreased articular cartilage in the weight-bearing joints. The bony outgrowths are known as *spurs*. The subcutaneous Heberden's nodes may be present. The fragmented bony pieces become loose in the joint space and are known as *"joint mice."*

OSTEOARTHRITIS

This degenerative joint disease (DJD) that has a premature onset, is *initiated* by: neurosensory defects, chronic articular trauma, pre-existing rheumatoid arthritis, and aging (NOT by asymptomatic multiple osteochondromatosis, nor by intake of calcium and phosphate). Heberden nodes = enlarged *distal interphalangeal joints*.

OSTEOPOROSIS

This is a metabolic bone disease that results in a decreased bone density—less than that needed for mechanical support. Osteoporosis may result in a *compression* fracture of the vertebra or hip. This usually happens after a sudden bending or other movement. It occurs in postmenopausal women or men usually above the age of 75. In the lab, the serum levels for calcium, phosphorus, and alkaline phosphatase are usually *normal*. There is a decrease in the bone mass. Treatment includes prevention of the loss of bone mass, and increasing the bone density. Estrogen and calcium supplement replacement decreases the rate of bone resorption in postmenopausal women. Exercise is very important to help decrease this loss of bone density and to avoid additional fractures.

MUSCULAR DYSTROPHY

Muscular dystrophy is a result of a defective gene that causes a deficiency of *dystrophin* (a muscle protein). It is associated with tendon and muscle contractures, cardiomyopathy, and mild mental retardation. Muscle weakness results from the hypertrophy and replacement of the muscle by fat and connective tissue. On lab examination, there is a large elevation of the muscle enzymes, creatine kinase (CK) and aldolase. EMG shows necrosis of muscle. Dystrophin *gene* mutations can be determined by cDNA probes. Eventually, the patient will develop respiratory failure and infections. Cardiomyopathy may complicate. Treatment includes physical therapy and stretching of the affected muscles. Prednisone has also been useful.

DUCHENNE'S MUSCULAR DYSTROPHY

Duchenne's muscular dystrophy results from a defective gene that causes a *deficiency* of *dystrophin* (NOT defective actin). Its inheritance is sex-linked, and is fairly common (1 out of 3,500 males). Variable segmental gene deletions, lead to frame shift and stop codon formation. As a child, there is weakness that gradually develops into death at about 20 years of age. The usual cause of death is *respiratory insufficiency*. It is associated with weakness and mild mental retardation.

PAGET'S DISEASE OF THE BONE

This disease occurs as osteolytic and osteoblastic activity of the bone (increased activity of BOTH osteo*blasts* and osteo*clasts*). This causes pathological fractures. There is an *increased* serum alkaline phosphatase activity. *Normal* calcium and phosphate levels. This may also cause cardiovascular decompensation.

BENIGN GIANT CELL TUMOR

Radiolucent tumor that expands the extremity of a long bone.

MULTIPLE MYELOMA

This is a plasma cell disorder and osteolytic (NOT osteoblastic) bone disease, and presents as a *malignant* increase of plasma cells in the bone marrow. Multiple myeloma is considered the most common malignant gammopathy. Look for marrow plasmacytosis, lytic bone lesions (bone *pain* is the major complaint), and an M component in the serum and urine. The M protein is mainly IgG and some IgA, and Bence Jones proteinuria can also be seen. Multiple myeloma is associated with increased urine and serum calcium (hypercalcemia), increased total serum globulin, and mild azotemia. Radiologic findings will show "punched out" lesions due to the osteolytic changes.

WALDENSTROM'S MACROGLOBULINEMIA

This is another malignant bone disease (lymphoplasmacytic) seen with the hypersecretion of IgM (the M protein). It is also associated with cryoglobulinemia in lower temperatures.

OSTEOMYELITIS

The most common agent causing osteomyelitis is *Staphylococcus aureus*. In diabetes mellitus the causative organism is *Salmonella*.

FIBROUS DYSPLASIA

This metaplasia is the replacement of bone with a fibrous mixture of woven bone. Leads to cortical expansion, may cause severe cosmetic deformity, incomplete maturation of bone. Fibrous dysplasia of bone associated with precocious puberty. (Does NOT increase serum alkaline phosphatase, does NOT develop malignant melanoma, does NOT form cartilaginous metaplasia of the bone.) (NOT premalignant)

OSTEOMALACIA

This is a disease in which the bones fail to calcify due to a deficiency of Vitamin D or kidney dysfunction. It is seen in adults as painful, softened bones (lack of calcification). "Bow-legged" and other deformities because of the failure of bone mineralization. In children, this is called *Rickets*. Osteopenia by X-Ray. Osteomalacia is very dangerous if the patient is pregnant. It is associated with renal osteodystrophy, normal or decreased serum calcium, decreased phosphate, and an *increased* alkaline phosphatase level (NOT increased PTH).

HYALINE

This is a glassy, homogenous pink appearing substance. It is found with thickened, homogenous, viral inclusions. It also deposits in hepatocytes of chronic alcoholics, and in chronic hypertension in the arteriolar basement membranes.

PROCALLUS

This is granulation tissue with islands of cartilage that bridges the site of a fracture.

WORKLOAD FOR SKELETAL MUSCLE

With an increased workload for skeletal muscle, changes include: increased number of mitochondria, increased number of myofilaments (increased number of *organelles*), and an increased number of sarcoplasmic reticulum (NOT an increased number of nuclei). Physiologic *hypertrophy* is an increase in the *size* of the muscle cells. (Remember, *hyperplasia* is the increase in the *number* of cells—for example, an increase in the number of liver cells. Hyperplasia does NOT occur in nerves, cardiac muscle, nor skeletal muscle.)

ANKYLOSING SPONDYLITIS

This is associated with **HLA B27**, male predominance, and osseous metaplasia. (It is NOT associated with: arthritis, urethritis, conjunctivitis, splenomegaly, polyarteritis, nor leukopenia.) It may lead to pulmonary insufficiency.

HLA-B27

This is associated with Ankylosing Spondylitis, Reiter's syndrome, and adult Rheumatoid Arthritis.

RHEUMATOID ARTHRITIS

This likely autoimmune disorder can cause destruction of the involved joints (enzymes like proteases and collagenases destroy the cartilage). Villous hypertrophy of the synovium with infiltration is considered *pannus formation*. Rheumatoid nodule lesions occur in subcutaneous tissue, lung, and heart (there are NO pathogenic organisms in the lesions). Rheumatoid factor forms in the joint fluid and neutrophils, lymphocytes, and other cells accumulate in the joint space.

RHEUMATOID FACTOR

Rheumatoid factor is an **IgM** antibody against the **Fc** portion of **IgG**.

GONOCOCCAL ARTHRITIS

This is a *suppurative* arthritis, and is seen as an inflammation of the synovium by bacterial invasion (usually of the large joints). For example, gonococcal arthritis may be seen in a teenaged patient who presents with a painful, red, and warm swollen *knee*. On examination of the synovial fluid, you will likely remove a cloudy, thin fluid with clots and PMNs.

TUBERCULOUS ARTHRITIS

This tuberculous osteomyelitis is seen in *Pott's disease* of the spine. It is more destructive than gonococcal or other suppurative arthritis.

GOUTY ARTHRITIS

This is hyperuricemia with a stage of purulent inflammation, and a stage of granuloma formation. *Tophaceous gout* is a chronic gout, with crystallized urates in the joints. (Gouty arthritis does NOT form "joint mice.")

Syndromes 11

NOTE: The following syndromes are commonly tested on your examinations. They are also clinically relevant in your future practice in medicine. In general, whenever you find one defect or genetic difference by physical examination, you should consider that the patient most likely has another defect (cardiovascular or other). This is why they are *syndromes*.

ADRENOGENITAL SYNDROME

This syndrome is associated with adrenocortical hyperplasia or malignant tumor, masculinization or feminization, precocious puberty, decreased plasma cortisol, and increased urinary 17-ketosteroids.

ADULT RESPIRATORY DISTRESS SYNDROME (ARDS)

ARDS includes alveolar and interstitial *edema*, and increased collagen fibers. The alveolar capillary damage develops into respiratory failure and hypoxemia. Loss of *surfactant* leads to atelectasis and pulmonary edema.

CARCINOID SYNDROME

Carcinoid tumors of the GI that release *serotonin*, and metastasize to the liver. Carcinoid tumors are most common in the ileum and appendix. Carcinoid syndrome is associated with: paroxysmal flushing, wheezing, *watery* diarrhea, skin lesions, and *right*-sided heart failure. Furthermore, check for *ileal* carcinoids and the metastasis to the liver.

BUDD-CHIARI SYNDROME

Budd-Chiari Syndrome is associated with: *thrombosis of hepatic vein*, hepatomegaly, portal hypertension and ascites, and thrombotic tendencies.

CHEDIAK-HIGASHI SYNDROME

This includes: oculocutaneous albinism, lysosomal defects, impaired chemotaxis, and recurrent infections.

CONN'S SYNDROME

This is due to an excess of mineralocorticoids. It is associated with: increased aldosterone—therefore, increased NaCl absorption and potassium excretion, hypernatremia, and decreased plasma renin. Also, increased potassium *excretion*, sodium *absorption*, and hypertension (NOT hyperkalemia, NOT metabolic acidosis).

CRI-DU-CHAT SYNDROME

This is a result of a partial deletion of the short arm of chromosome 5 (as 46 XX 5p–) or (46 XY 5p–) occurring at a normal maternal age, and appears as microcephaly, retardation, and a high-pitched cry (like a cat).

CRIGLER-NAJJAR SYNDROME

This autosomal recessive syndrome appears as the inability to form adequate bilirubin glucuronide, jaundice. There is a decrease or absence of UDP-glucoronyl transferase, and therefore no conjugation of bilirubin. The result is an increase in **un**conjugated bilirubin.

CUSHING'S SYNDROME

This syndrome appears as a *pituitary* hypersecretion of *ACTH*. It may be due to a tumor or adrenocortical hyperplasia, or to exogenous steroids. There is an *increased* plasma *cortisol*, urine 17-hydroxy corticosteroids and free cortisol. *Pituitary*-based hypercortisolism is Cushing's *disease*. This hypercortisolism (with an increased ACTH) can be suppressed by HIGH doses of dexamethasone. There are *decreased* urinary 17-hydroxy corticosteroids *as a response to* HIGH dose of dexamethasone (suppression results from HIGH not low dose). If it is an *ectopic* ACTH production, then the cortisol production will NOT be suppressed by high dose dexamethasone. Furthermore, a loss of diurnal variation of plasma cortisol occurs in Cushing's. Cushing's is associated with: central obesity, hypertension, osteoporosis, abdominal stria, "moon face," glucose intolerance, and polycythemia.

DANDY-WALKER SYNDROME

Dandy-Walker syndrome includes: infantile hydrocephalus, and atresia of the Foramen of Magendi.

DOWN'S SYNDROME

Down's syndrome is characterized by: trisomy 21, mental retardation, flat face, palmar simian crease, epicanthal folds, and a large protruding tongue (Fig. 11-1). Down's syndrome is associated with an increased incidence of congestive heart disease, acute leukemia, and Alzheimer's disease. Nondisjunction is the cause of approximately 95% of the cases of Down's and is due to an additional chromosome 21 (47, XY, +21). 4% of cases are due to Robertsonian translocation with the long arm of 21 onto 22 or 14 [46, XX, −14, +t(14q, 21q)]. The other approximately 1% are considered *mosaics*, and have mixed normal cells (46) and cells with an extra chromosome 21 (47). In mothers of age greater than 45 years old, there is a 1 in 25 chance of developing a child with Down's (increasing risk with maternal age over 35).

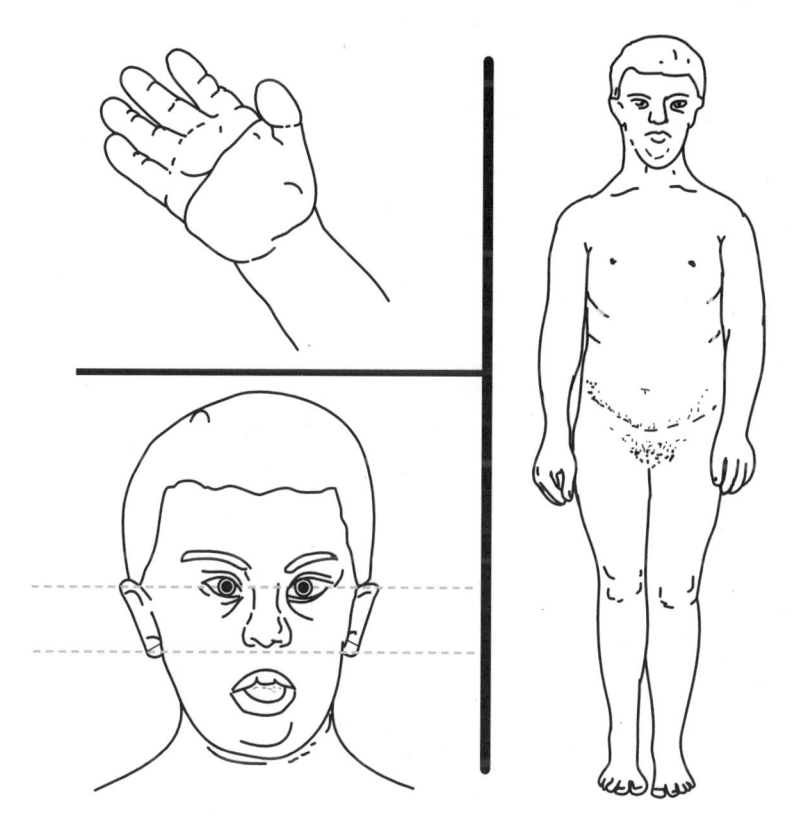

Figure 11-1 Down's Syndrome. Characteristics include: *Hands:* short middle phalanx of fingers and short hands, simian crease (single palmar crease); *Facial features:* broad nasal bridge, epicanthal folds, wide-spaced eyes, low-set ears, large protruding tongue, Brushfield's spots (peripheral white spots of iris); *Body:* short stature, hyperflexibility, congenital heart disease (ventricular septal defects), susceptibility to infection, pelvic abnormalities, brain changes similar to Alzheimer's disease.

DUBIN-JOHNSON SYNDROME

This is a cause of chronic jaundice seen with *conjugated* hyperbilirubinemia. It is associated with a darkly pigmented liver, and is considered benign.

EDWARD'S SYNDROME

This syndrome is caused by an extra chromosome 18 or Trisomy **18** (47 XX +18 for the female, or 47 XY +18 for the male). Edward's is associated with: mental retardation, micrognathia, low set ears, flexible fingers, *rocker-bottom feet*, and *horseshoe kidney*.

FANCONI'S SYNDROME

This inherited syndrome affects children, and appears as anemia, acidosis, skeletal problems and decreased renal tubular function (proximal renal tubule dysfunction). It is associated with multiple myeloma, glycosuria, and systemic acidosis.

GARDNER'S SYNDROME

Multiple tumors of the skull, epidermis and fibromas. There is an increased occurrence of polyposis and cancer of the colon.

GILBERT'S SYNDROME

This is the most common hereditary hyperbilirubinemia. Familial jaundice, with increased serum **un**conjugated bilirubin. In Gilbert's syndrome, the **un**conjugated bilirubin will increase because of the lack of conversion to the conjugated bilirubin.

GOODPASTURE'S SYNDROME

Goodpasture's is identified by immunoglobulin deposits that form crescents on the ***alveolar*** and the ***glomerular*** *basement membranes* (anti-glomerular basement membrane antibodies). It has a linear immunofluorescent pattern of Ig**G** (NOT IgE). There is a rapid decrease in the *renal* function, and *pulmonary* hemorrhage may occur.

GUILLAIN-BARRÉ SYNDROME

This is an acute, "ascending" neuropathy that occurs following an infection (like CMV, EBV) or other event (trauma). Polyneuritis with radicular demyelination may occur. It presents as a *myalgia* and weakness, with possible bilateral facial weakness (paralysis) and ophthalmoplegia. Usually the patients will recover completely, and treatment is supportive.

HORNER'S SYNDROME

This includes: ptosis, anhidrosis (no sweating), and miosis.

HUNTER'S SYNDROME

Also known as Type **II** mucopolysaccharidosis and Gargoylism, as a result of *sulfatase* deficiency. There is an increased urinary excretion of chondroitin sulfate and heparin sulfate (the cornea is NOT cloudy).

HURLER'S SYNDROME

Also known as Type **I** mucopolysaccharidosis, as a result of α-*L*-*iduronidase* deficiency. There is an increased urinary excretion of chondroitin sulfate and heparin sulfate. It forms very abnormal cartilage, Gargoylism, and a *cloudy cornea*.

KIMMELSTIEL-WILSON SYNDROME

This syndrome is seen with diabetes mellitus, and is associated with hypertension, proteinuria, and edema.

KLINEFELTER'S SYNDROME

This syndrome is the result of a 47, XXY genotype (extra X chromosomes). Klinefelter's patient is a *male* with seminiferous tubule dysgenesis, and increased urine gonadotropins. It is associated with: tall stature, small hypoplastic testes, male infertility, one Y chromosome and more than one X chromosome, testicular atrophy, eunuchoid body habitus, gynecomastia, and female distribution of hair. This can be demonstrated by a chromatin-positive buccal smear (a male individual with a Barr body).

LEIGH'S SYNDROME

This is considered an autosomal recessive syndrome characterized by subacute necrotizing encephalomyelopathy. The brain lesions are **bi**lateral, and there is a decrease in cytochrome C oxidase or pyruvate dehydrogenase.

LESCH-NYHAN SYNDROME

This is an X-linked recessive syndrome that results from hypoxanthine-guanine phosphoribosyl transferase (HGPRT) deficiency. It is only seen in *males*, and is associated with hyperuricemia, choreoathetosis, compulsive self-mutilation, and mental retardation.

MALLORY-WEISS SYNDROME

Lower esophageal lesion, causes bleeding or penetrates to the mediastinum, and is associated with *vomiting*. Remember, the linear tears of the esophageal lumen are caused by vomiting and a problem with the relaxation reflex of the LES. Therefore, it is mostly seen in *alcoholics*.

MARFAN'S SYNDROME

This is an autosomal *dominant* connective tissue disease. It is associated with: tall stature, arachnodactyly (long "spider" fingers), joint hyperextension, pectus excavatum, iridodonesis (iris lacks support from lens), ectopia lentis (dislocation of the lens), "floppy valve syndrome" with aortic and mitral valve abnormalities, and eventual dissecting aortic aneurysm (it is NOT associated with hepatocellular carcinoma). This is probably the only disease related to the age of the *father* (usually the father was over 65 years old at the time of conception of the patient).

MEIG'S SYNDROME

Triad: Ovarian tumor, ascites, and hydrothorax.

PANCOAST SYNDROME

This syndrome is associated with: constricted pupil, levator palpebra superioris muscle paralysis, and a malignant tumor. It also is associated with pain and tingles in the arm of the affected ulnar nerve.

PATAU'S SYNDROME

This is Trisomy **13** (47 XX +13 in the female or 47 XY +13 in the male). It is associated with: *microcephaly*, mental retardation, microphthalmia, *cleft lip and palate, polydactyly*, ventricular septal defect, and cardiac *dextroposition* (the heart is on the *right* side).

PEUTZ-JEGHERS SYNDROME

This is an autosomal *dominant* syndrome that is associated with: multiple polyposis of the GI (the *jejunum* is most affected), and freckles on the lips (melanin spots).

REITER'S SYNDROME

Triad: Urethritis, iridocyclitis (conjunctivitis), and arthritis.

REYE'S SYNDROME

Reye's syndrome occurs with children treated with *aspirin* for a viral infection that may produce a sudden loss of consciousness, cerebral edema, *fatty change to the liver* and kidney, and possibly death.

SANFILIPPO'S SYNDROME

This is an autosomal recessive syndrome, also known as Type **III** mucopolysaccharidosis. An accumulation of heparan sulfate is caused by the deficiency of *heparan N-sulfatase*. It results in severe mental retardation, and hepatomegaly.

SÉZARY SYNDROME

This includes exfoliative dermatitis, pruritis, and is associated with alopecia, and edema. The "Sézary" cells have a cerebriform nucleus, and this is associated with a T-cell origin and leukemia.

SHEEHAN'S SYNDROME

Hypopituitarism from *postpartum pituitary necrosis* (from obstetric hemorrhage). It often results in partial loss of pituitary mass, inability to lactate, and may lead to ischemic injury of 95% of the anterior pituitary.

SIPPLE'S SYNDROME

This is an autosomal dominant syndrome and is considered a Multiple endocrine neoplasia syndrome (MEN type II). It is associated with: pheochromocytoma, medullary thyroid carcinoma, and parathyroid adenomas.

SIDS (SUDDEN INFANT DEATH SYNDROME)

This is diagnosed by exclusion, and is considered "crib death." It is the sudden, unexpected death of a previously healthy infant, and the cause of death is unexplained—even by autopsy. Increased risk factors include: premature, low birth weight, sleeping on stomach, and previous history of SIDS in sibling.

SJÖGREN'S SYNDROME

Sjögren's syndrome is associated with: keratoconjunctivitis, dry mouth, telangiectasias, bilaterally enlarged parotid glands, and lymphocytic infiltration of the lacrimal gland, with *decreased* salivation. It is *more* common than SLE, but *less* common than Rheumatoid Arthritis.

STEIN-LEVANTHAL SYNDROME

This is a syndrome that presents as: infertility, obesity, amenorrhea, (menstrual abnormalities), hirsutism (hairy), and **bi**laterally enlarged *polycystic ovaries*.

TURNER'S SYNDROME (Fig. 11-2)

45,XO Aneuploidy that presents as: short stature, small fibrotic "streak ovaries," webbed neck, wide-spaced nipples, broad chest, pigmented nevi, NO Barr bodies, female phenotype, amenorrhea, infantile genitalia (infertility), and an increased incidence of coarctation of the aorta (NOT an increase in estrogen, and NOT a decrease in hCG).

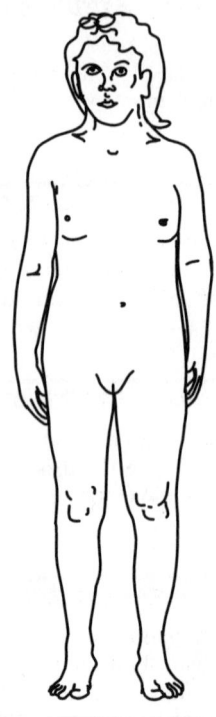

Figure 11-2 Turner's Syndrome. Characteristics include: micrognathia and enlarged ears, webbed neck, poorly developed genitalia, short stature, wide-spaced nipples and broad chest, primary amenorrhea, congenital heart disease, and fibrous/atrophic ovaries.

WATERHOUSE-FRIDERICHSEN SYNDROME

This is most commonly due to *Neisseria meningococcal* septicemia. It presents as vomiting, diarrhea, vascular collapse, and convulsions. Waterhouse-Friderichsen syndrome is a severe adrenal insufficiency that is due to hemorrhagic necrosis of the adrenal cortex.

Miscellaneous   12

SERUM HCG

Human **c**horionic **g**onadotropin is *increased* in: ovarian carcinoma, choriocarcinoma, hydatidiform mole, trophoblastic disease, testicular germ cell tumor (testicular carcinoma) (NOT Stein-Levanthal Syndrome). (NOT carcinoma of the endometrium, NOT colo-rectal cancer, and NOT from pituitary tumor.)

α-1-FETOPROTEIN

This tumor marker is used to monitor progression of *hepatocellular carcinoma*. It is *increased* in:
    hepatocellular carcinoma (hepatoma),
    malignant teratoma of the ovary, and
    yolk sac tumors

(NOT small cell carcinoma of the lung, NOT colorectal cancer, NOT with metastatic bronchogenic carcinoma, NOT with metastatic melanoma, and NOT choriocarcinoma).

AFLATOXIN B1

This is considered a chemical carcinogen that induces hepatocellular carcinomas.

BRUTON'S TYPE AGAMMAGLOBULINEMIA

This is an inherited (X-linked) disorder that usually affects males and is diagnosed after 6 months of age. This condition results in recurrent *bacterial* infections (*Staph.*, and *H. influenzae*). There are NO B-cells and therefore, NO serum immunoglobulin. (CMI is normal with T cells present.) These patients retain the ability for homograft rejections, acute inflammation, and delayed cutaneous hypersensitivity. But, they will NOT have *active* immunization (i.e., by tetanus toxoid).

CHRONIC LEAD POISONING

Lead poisoning is associated with basophilic *stippling* of the red blood cells, anemia, increased urine porphyrins, and δ-amino levulinic acid (ALA) in the urine.

CONSIDERED PRECANCEROUS LESIONS

Bowen's disease, Erythroplasia of Queyrat, actinic keratosis, solar keratosis of the skin, lentigo maligna, chronic atrophic gastritis, leukoplakia of vulva and penis, familial polyposis coli (NOT verruca wart).

FREE RADICALS

Free radicals can be generated by deposits of lipofuscin pigments, from phagocytosis of microorganisms, and from carbon tetrachloride toxicity (NOT from cyanide poisoning).

EPIDURAL HEMATOMA

This is a hematoma that results from a ruptured *meningeal artery* that increases the intracranial pressure, and occurs between the *skull and dura*. It usually occurs after a skull *fracture*.

SUBDURAL HEMATOMA

This is a hematoma that results from ruptured *bridging veins*, and occurs between the *dura and arachnoid*. It usually occurs after trauma and to *alcoholics* (after they black out and fall to hit their head).

LABORATORY TECHNIQUES

Allele specific oligonucleotide hybridization—detects single nucleotide change in known gene.
Polymerase chain reaction—analyzes minute clinical samples.
RFLP (Restriction Fragment Length Polymorphisms)—genetic linkage analysis.
Southern blot—restriction endonucleases digests, then electrophoresis, transfer and hybridization with a probe.
Guthrie test—used for the early detection of PKU (phenylketonuria).

TAY-SACHS DISEASE

Metabolic disorder of *ganglioside*, it is a deficiency of hexosaminidase A enzyme, and is common among individuals with Jewish ancestry. On exam, the

GM_2-ganglioside will be elevated. It is associated with *cherry-red spot* in the retina. This lysosomal storage disease usually results in death by 2 or 3 years of age.

GAUCHER'S DISEASE

Lysosomal storage disease that results in increased glucocerebrosides (ceramide) due to a deficiency of *glucocerebrosidase*. Look for PAS positive Gaucher's cells and the "crumpled tissue paper" appearance. It is associated with interstitial lung disease, hepatosplenomegaly, and hemolytic anemia. Adults (type I) and children (type II for infants, and type III is *less* severe) have different forms. Gaucher's cells are large histiocytes.

NEIMANN-PICK DISEASE

Increased sphingomyelin due to a deficiency of sphingomyelinase.

VON GIERKE'S DISEASE

This is a glycogen storage disease that results from a deficiency of *glucose-6-phosphatase*. This results in an increase of glycogen and a decrease of glucose.

McARDLE'S DISEASE

This glycogen storage disease results from a deficiency of *muscle phosphorylase* that leads to an increase in glycogen and muscle cramps and weakness.

POMPE'S DISEASE

This results from a deficiency of *acid maltase* (α-glucosidase) that leads to storage of glycogen in the *heart*. Finally, cardiomegaly and death.

PSEUDOMYXOMA PERITONEI

May be caused by mucocele of the appendix.

HOMOZYGOUS HEMOGLOBIN C DISEASE

This presents as mild hemolytic anemia, splenomegaly, intraerythrocytic crystals, and β-chains of hemoglobin have a single amino acid substitution (NOT numerous tear drop cells—which are seen in *myelofibrosis* and *thalassemia*).

EBSTEIN BARR VIRUS (EBV)

EBV is associated with *Burkitt's lymphoma*, infectious mononucleosis, and nasopharyngeal carcinoma.

CYTOMEGALOVIRUS (CMV)

This virus usually affects immunocompromised individuals, and infects the liver cells as *inclusion bodies* with a surrounding halo. Therefore, on microscopic examination, look for enlarged cells—that appear like an "**owl's eye**."

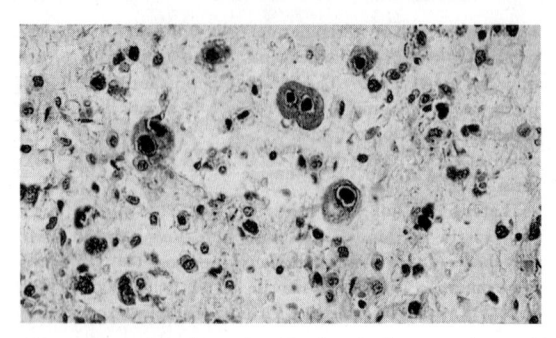

Figure 12-1 Cytomegalovirus Inclusion Bodies. Pulmonary intracellular inclusion bodies from a CMV infection. The large intranuclear inclusions and surrounding halo create the "owl's eye" appearance. (For a color version see Color Plate 24.)

HIV AND AIDS

Human immunodeficiency virus (HIV) is transmitted and enters the body from blood or body secretions, and affects the immune system. It attacks the lymphocytes with the CD4 surface receptors (T helper cells). This leads to infection and destruction of the T helper cells and increased infections to other opportunists (fungi, bacteria, parasites and viruses). This is associated with subacute encephalopathy, and contains multinucleated giant cells (CMV infection). To diagnose, *first* test the patient's serum by the ELISA method for the serum antibody. If the result is positive, then the second test to *confirm* the result with a very specific test is the Western Blot technique.

At CD4 counts below 500 cells, Azidothymidine (AZT) and other combination drug therapies have been used to slow the progression of a HIV infection to AIDS. At CD4 counts below 200 cells, *Pneumocystis carinii* prophylaxis (TMP/SMX) is usually given with Acyclovir. Immunizations like pneumovax, influenza B, and hepatitis B are also part of the management. (NO intranuclear eosinophilic or basophilic inclusions.) AIDS usually occurs following 5–10 years of infection with HIV virus. HIV infection develops into AIDS when there is an *opportunistic infection* and a low CD4 count.

HEALING BY SECOND INTENTION

(Different from first by:) Quantitative use of granulation tissue, epithelial gap bridged by granulation tissue. Extensive necrotic tissue and exudate. It results from rapid epithelial closure (it does NOT involve specific cellular components).

RABIES

Associated with: *negri bodies*, hydrophobia, and is almost always fatal (it is NOT a subclinical infection).

HEMOPHILUS INFLUENZA

This can be found in a child with severe headache, fever, and stiff neck for hours. The Cerebral Spinal Fluid usually has many of these extracellular *gram negative bacilli*.

RADIATION SICKNESS

After whole body radiation, you will see *nausea and vomiting* first.

DEHYDRATION

Dehydration causes an increased serum albumin concentration, and increases BUN and Creatinine.

AUTOSOMAL RECESSIVE

Autosomal *recessive* diseases are usually most of the *enzyme deficiencies*. Examples of autosomal recessive diseases include: Gaucher's disease, Niemann-Pick's disease, Hurler's Syndrome, and Cystic fibrosis.

X-LINKED INHERITANCE

A few conditions that are X-linked include: *Hunter's* Syndrome, Lesch-Nyhan Syndrome, G6PD deficiency, and Fabry's Disease.

STAINING

Perform *tissue stain* for fungi and acid-fast bacilli. Perform *Gram stain* for bacteria, and microscopy under polarized light.

GLUCOCORTICOSTEROIDS

These have an effect on the inflammatory process by: inhibiting phospholipase A_2 used for arachidonic acid synthesis, causing membrane stabilization of lysosomes, and inhibiting vasodilation. (They do NOT inhibit the cyclo-oxygenase path of prostaglandin synthesis).

LIPOMAS

These are usually *solitary* masses of fatty tissue that originates from mesenchymal *lipocytes*. The lipoma fat is NOT available for usage by the body. It is a benign mass that can be excised if desired (it is NOT premalignant).

$$\textbf{SPECIFICITY} = \frac{\text{True } Negative}{\text{True } Negative + \text{False } Positive}$$

Those who tested *negative* (and therefore do *not* have the disease), divided by all those without the disease. It determines how effective your test is at finding the people who are well (no disease).

$$\textbf{SENSITIVITY} = \frac{\text{True } Positive}{\text{True } Positive + \text{False } Negative}$$

Those who tested *positive* (and therefore have the disease), divided by all those with the disease. It determines how well you identify people *with* the disease. It is usually the *first* test used, like a screening test when there are public health threats (i.e., TB, polio, or meningitis).

FALSE NEGATIVE

When a test reports a negative result and the person actually *has* the disease.

FALSE POSITIVE

When a test reports a positive result, and the person actually does NOT have the disease.

$$\textbf{POSITIVE PREDICTIVE VALUE} = \frac{\text{True } Positives}{\text{True Positives + False Positives}}$$

True positives divided by all persons testing positive. Determines the percentage of people that *have* the disease, out of those who tested *positive*.

$$\textbf{NEGATIVE PREDICTIVE VALUE} = \frac{\text{True } Negatives}{\text{True Negatives + False Negatives}}$$

True negatives divided by all persons testing negative. Determines the percentage of people that do NOT have the disease, out of those who tested *negative*. This gives you the *chance* that the person does NOT have the disease.

EFFICIENCY OF LAB TEST RESULT

True *negative* and true *positive* test results which would come from the total population of *healthy and diseased* people tested.

CREATININE CLEARANCE

This gives an estimation of the glomerular filtration rate (GFR).

$$\text{Cr. Cl} = \frac{(140 - \text{age})(\text{wt in kg})}{72 \times (\text{Serum Cr in mg/dL})} \text{ for men}$$

for women (multiply result by 0.85)

SERUM CREATININE

Lab test showing decreased renal *function*

$$\text{Serum } \frac{\text{Urea}}{\text{Creatinine}} \text{ ratio} > 15 = \text{Prerenal or postrenal azotemia}$$

$$\text{MCV} = \frac{\text{Hct}}{\text{RBC}} \times 10$$

The mean corpuscular volume is usually around **87** (and the volume is considered to be normo**cytic**).

$$\text{MCH} = \frac{\text{Hb}}{\text{RBC}} \times 10$$

The MCH is usually around **30**.

$$\text{MCHC} = \frac{\text{Hb}}{\text{Hct}} \times 10$$

The MCHC is usually around **33** to be considered normo**chromic**.

"Cancer"	"Most Common . . ."
Malignant Melanoma	Most common skin cancer in a younger patient.
Squamous cell carcinoma	Most common malignant tumor of the oral cavity.
	(continued)

(Continued)

"Cancer"	"Most Common . . ."
Pleomorphic adenoma	Most common salivary gland tumor.
Parotid gland	Most common area of salivary gland tumors.
Carcinoid tumors	Most common location is in the ileum and the appendix.
Glioblastoma multiforme	Most common *glioma* in *adults*. Most common primary intracranial neoplasm.
Wilm's tumor of the kidney	Most common in children 2–4 yrs. old.
***Papillary* thyroid cancer**	Most common thyroid cancer.
Prolactinoma	Most common pituitary gland neoplasm. (Most common of all pituitary adenomas.)
Chromophobic cell adenomas	Most common *non*-secretory pituitary adenomas.
1. Cerebellar Astrocytoma **2. Medulloblastoma**	Most common posterior fossa tumor in *Children*. (located midline cerebellar)
Myxoma	Most common heart tumor.
Osteosarcoma	Most common tumor of the bone.
Fibroadenoma	Most common *benign* tumor of the breast.
Leiomyoma	Most common neoplasm of the uterus.
Fibrocystic disease of the breast	Most common breast lesion in women.
Bronchogenic Carcinoma (lung cancer)	Most common cause of cancer death in males and females.
Multiple myeloma	Most common malignant gammopathy.

Chemical Carcinogen Exposure	Associated Carcinoma
Tobacco, Aniline dyes, Rubber products	Papillary carcinoma of the urinary bladder (Transitional cell CA)
Asbestos	Mesothelioma of the pleura
DES	Clear cell carcinoma of the vagina in child of mother who used DES.
Vinyl chloride (plastics), Arsenic, Thorotrast	Hemangiosarcoma of the liver

Tumor Marker	Associated Cancer
CEA (Carcinoembryonic antigen)	Used to monitor therapy of *colorectal carcinoma.*
S-100 protein	Melanoma; neural tumors.
AFP (α-fetoprotein)	Germ cell tumors; Primary liver cancers
PSA	Prostatic carcinoma
CA–125	Ovarian tumors

ENVIRONMENTAL PATHOLOGY

Be aware that the *environment* plays a crucial role in the development of pathology in the body. Tissue injury can occur from frostbite, hypothermia, heat stroke, burns, electrical injury, radiation, air pollutants, asbestos, and other agents. Tobacco, alcohol, marijuana, heroin, cocaine, carbon monoxide, cyanide, heavy metals (lead, mercury, and others), and medications can alter the body systems and tissues. Cyanide induces cell death by *inactivating cytochrome oxidase.*

Memorize the following associations:

Carbon monoxide	Increased hemoglobin affinity
Cyanide	Bitter almond breath (odor)

(continued)

(Continued)	
Methanol	Blindness
Asbestos	Asbestos bodies, Pleural calcifications, *Mesothelioma*
Silica dust	Silicosis, with fibrotic changes, Increased risk for TB

The graph below is very important to understand. For the graph, try to clinically correlate the concepts of calcium levels with PTH levels for certain diseases. Notice that the PTH elevates as you go up, and the calcium increases as you go to the right. As you learn the different disorders, then apply them to the graph and that is the location for your answer.

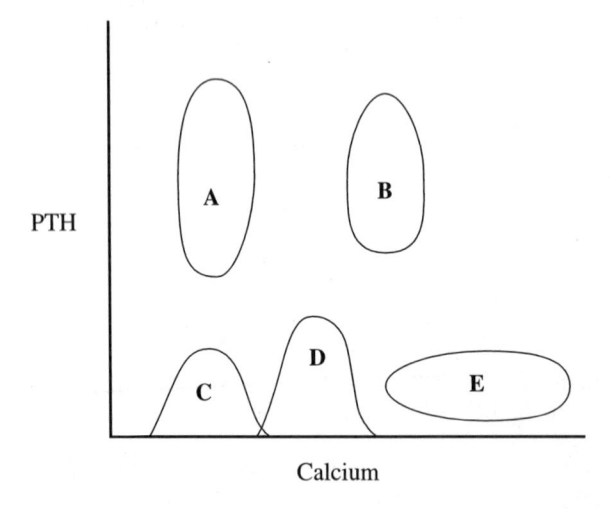

A would be Chronic renal failure. This is due to the decreased Vitamin D and decreased calcium which increases PTH. This is considered *secondary* hyperparathyroidism.

B would be **Hyper**parathyroidism. This is due to the increased PTH level and this increases the calcium level (decreases phosphate and increases alkaline phosphatase). It is also seen in other bone diseases.

C would be **Hypo**parathyroidism. This is due to the *decreased* PTH level and therefore, the decreased calcium (and increased phosphate).

D would be the Normal individual.

E would be Multiple myeloma. This is due to the increased calcium level (from bone resorption) and therefore, decreased PTH.

Remember, PTH *increases* the calcium level, and calcitonin *decreases* the calcium level. Also, a *decrease* in vitamin D will cause PTH to *increase*.

Congratulations, you have completely reviewed the essentials of pathology with Digging Up the Bones®. *You have the important topics and concepts that are heavily tested on your exams. Now, I would like to wish you continued success in the future, because you have the knowledge to do well. Please write and let me know how you did and if we can add or change things in the future. Best wishes!*

Index

Index

A

Abetalipoproteinemia, 47
Abruptio placenta, 84
Achalasia, 42
Acoustic neuroma, 68
Acromegaly, 65
Acute bronchitis, 50
Acute cholecystitis, 78
Acute glomerular nephritis, 73–74
Acute lymphoblastic leukemia, 17
Acute myeloblastic leukemia, 17
Acute myocardial infarction, 27
Acute pyelonephritis, 79
Acute renal failure, 75–76
Acute tubular necrosis, 76
Addison's disease, 59
Adenocarcinoma in cecum, 46
Adenocarcinoma of lung, 53
Adrenal glands, 59–62
Adrenal medulla tumors, 61
Adrenogenital syndrome, 97
Adult respiratory distress syndrome (ARDS), 56, 97
Aflatoxin B1, 105
Agammaglobulinemia, 105
AIDS, 108
Alcohol abuse, 38
Alcoholic cirrhosis, 38
Alkaline phosphatase, 92
Alzheimer's disease, 70
Amyloblastoma, 65
Amyloid, 21
Amyloidosis, 21–22
Amyotrophic lateral sclerosis (ALS), 91
Anemia, 18–19, 42
Anion gap, 25
Ankylosing spondylitis, 96

Antemortem thrombus, 33
Anterior pituitary insufficiency, 61
α-1-antitrypsin deficiency, 38
APTT (activated partial thromboplastin time), 11
APUD tumors, 61
ARDS (adult respiratory distress syndrome), 56, 97
Asbestosis, 55
Ascites, 9
Ascorbic acid (Vitamin C), 4, 6
Ascorbic acid deficiency, 4, 6
Aspirin, 12
Atherosclerosis, 31
Atrial septal defect (ASD), 29
Atrophic chronic gastritis, 42, 43
Atypical pneumonia, 51
Autosomal recessive, 109
Azotemia, 76

B

Bacterial pneumonia, 51
Basal cell carcinoma, 85–86
Basophils, 8
Benign neoplasia, 54
Benign prostatic hypertrophy (BPH), 82
Berger's disease, 74
Berry aneurysms, 78
β-thalassemia, 19
Black lung disease, 54
Bleeding time, 11
Bowen's disease, 86
Bradykinin, 9
Breast carcinoma, 88–90
Breast mass, 87

Bronchial asthma, 57
Bronchial carcinoid, 54
Bronchiectasis, 57
Bronchioloalveolar carcinoma, 53
Bronchitis, 50, 52
Bronchogenic carcinomas, 53, 112
Brown atrophy of heart, 32
Bruton's type agammaglobulinemia, 105–106
Budd-Chiari syndrome, 37, 97
Burkitt's lymphoma, 15, 16

C

Calcification, 14
Calcitonin, 63
Carcinogenic promoters, 1
Carcinoid syndrome, 45, 97
Carcinoid tumors, 112
Carcinoma of breast, 88–90
Carcinoma of cervix, 81
Carcinoma of esophagus, 41
Carcinoma of gallbladder, 36
Carcinoma of larynx, 55
Carcinoma of lung, 52–53, 112
Carcinoma of prostate, 82
Carcinoma of stomach, 43
CEA (carcinoembryonic antigen), 113
Celiac disease, 45
Cell injury, 13
Cell ischemia, 21
Cellular anoxia, 21
Centrilobular emphysema, 52
Chalones, 2
Chediak-Higashi syndrome, 97
Chemotactic agents, 7
Cholelithiasis (gallstones), 36
Chondrosarcoma, 91–92
Choriocarcinoma, 81
Christmas disease (Hemophilia B), 10, 11
Chromophobic cell adenomas, 112
Chromosomal translocation, 16
Chronic gastritis, 42

Chronic bronchitis, 50, 52
Chronic granulocytic leukemia, 18
Chronic granulomatous disease of childhood, 21
Chronic granulomatous inflammation, 18
Chronic ischemia, 21
Chronic lead poisoning, 106
Chronic lymphocytic leukemia, 18
Chronic obstructive pulmonary disease (COPD), 51–52
Chronic prostatitis, 82
Cirrhosis of liver, 37–38
Cirrhotic liver, 37–38
Classic hemophilia, 10, 11
Colitis, 44
Collagen, 27
Colon cancer, 46
Compound nevus, 85
Congenital hydrocephalus, 69
Congenital lactose intolerance, 46
Congenital megacolon, 44
Congestive heart failure, 30
Conn's syndrome, 59–60, 98
Contact inhibition, 1
Craniopharyngioma, 68
Creatine kinase, 27
Creatinine clearance, 111
Cri-du-chat syndrome, 98
Crigler-Najjar syndrome, 37, 98
Crohn's disease, 44
Cryptorchidism, 81
Cushing's disease, 60
Cushing's syndrome, 60, 98
Cyanide, 113
Cyanosis, 30
Cyclooxygenase pathway, 12
Cystic fibrosis, 43, 50
Cytomegalovirus, 108

D

Dandy-Walker syndrome, 98
Degenerative joint disease (DJD), 93

Dehydration, 109
Diabetes insipidus, 60
Diabetes mellitus, 65–66
Diabetic ketoacidosis, 66
DIC (disseminated intravascular coagulation), 10
Diethylstilbestrol (DES), 84
Direct Coombs' test, 20
Dissecting aortic aneurysm, 31
Disseminated intravascular coagulation (DIC), 13
Diverticular disease of the colon, 47
Down's syndrome, 98–99
Drug addicts, 28
Dubin-Johnson syndrome, 37, 99
Duchenne's muscular dystrophy, 94
Ductal carcinoma, 88–89
Duodenal peptic ulcers, 43
Duodenal ulcer, 43
Dysphagia, 41
Dystrophic calcification, 14

E

Epstein-Barr virus, 15, 107
Ecchymoses, 2
Ectopic pregnancy, 83
Edema, inflammatory, 9
Edward's syndrome, 99
Embolism, 31–32
Emphysema, 52
Endocarditis, 28
Endometrial adenocarcinoma, 81
Endometriosis, 82
Epidural hematoma, 106
Epinephric diverticulum, 42
Ewing's sarcoma, 92
Exocrine pancreas, 35
Exudates, 22–23

F

Fabry's disease, 109
Factor IX, 10

Factor IX deficiency, 10
Factor VII, 10
Factor VIIIc, 10
Fanconi's syndrome, 100
α-1-Fetoprotein, 105
Fibroadenoma of breast, 88, 112
Fibrocystic disease of breast, 87, 112
Fibrous dysplasia, 95
Folate, 5
Folate deficiency, 4
Folic acid deficiency, 4
Free radicals, 106
Free thyroxin index, 64

G

G6PD deficiency, 19
α-Galactosidase A deficiency, 109
Gallbladder, 36
Gallstones, 36
Gangrene, 65
Gardner's syndrome, 100
Gastric peptic ulcers, 42
Gastritis, 42–43
Gaucher's disease, 107
Generalized edema, 000
GFR (glomerular filtration rate), 111
Ghon's lesion, 51
GI tract, 46
Giant cell, 9
Giant cell tumor, 94
Gilbert's syndrome, 37, 100
Glioblastoma multiforme, 65, 68, 112
Glomerulonephritis, 73, 74
Glucocorticosteroids, 109
Gohn complex, 50
Goiter, 63
Gonococcal arthritis, 96
Goodpasture's syndrome, 56, 100
Gout, 65
Gouty arthritis, 96
Granulation tissue, 23
Granuloma, 21

Granulomatous response, 21
Granulosa cell tumor, 80
Grave's disease, 63
Guaiac test, 46
Guillain-Barré syndrome, 100
Guthrie test, 106

H

Hageman factor, 7, 10
Hashimoto's thyroiditis, 62
Healing by second intention, 108
Hemangiosarcoma of liver, 40
Hemoglobin C disease, 19, 107
Hemolytic disease of newborn, 20
Hemophilus influenzae, 109
Hemorrhagic necrosis, 13, 14
Hemosiderin, 20
Heparan sulfate, 13
Hepatitis, 38–40
Hepatitis B virus, 39
Hepatocellular carcinoma, 40, 105
Hereditary nephritis, 74
Hereditary spherocytosis, 20
Hexosaminidase A, 106
Histamine, 9
Histiocytes, 8
Histiocytomas, 2
Histoplasmosis, 51
HIV, 108
HIV infections, 68–69
HLA B27, 96
Hodgkin's disease, 15
Holoprosencephaly, 68
Horner's syndrome, 100
Hunter's syndrome, 100
Huntington's disease, 68
Hurler's syndrome, 101
Hyaline, 95
Hyaline membrane disease, 95
Hydrothorax, 56
11-Hydroxylase deficiency, 62
17-Hydroxylase deficiency, 62
21-Hydroxylase deficiency, 61

Hyperaldosteronism, 59–60
Hyperbilirubinemia, 36–37
Hypercorticism, 61
Hyperlipoproteinemia type IIb, 000
Hyperparathyroidism, 64, 114
Hypersplenism, 40–41
Hypertension, 29
Hyperthyroidism, 63
Hyperuricemia, 76
Hypoparathyroidism, 64, 114
Hypothyroidism, primary, 63
Hypopituitarism, 61
Hyposplenism, 41
Hypovitaminosis D, 93
Hypoxia, 57

I

Idiopathic hemochromatosis, 35–36
IgA, 74
IgG, 8, 38, 39
IgM, 38, 39, 74
Increased hCG, 105
Infiltrating ductal carcinoma, 88
Inflammation, 7–8
Inflammatory bowel disease, 44
Interstitial nephritis, 74
Intestinal malabsorption, 45
Intestinal strangulation, 46
Intraabdominal hernia, 46
Intraductal papilloma, 88
Intrinsic factor, 11, 42
Intrinsic pathway, 11
Intussusception, 46
Involucrum, 93
Iodine deficiency, 63
Iron deficiency, 18

J

Junctional nevus, 85
Juvenile onset diabetes mellitus, 66

K

Kartagener's syndrome, 56
Kimmelstiel-Wilson syndrome, 101
Klinefelter's syndrome, 101
Kruckenberg's tumor, 47
Kwashiorkor, 45

L

Laboratory techniques, 106
Lead poisoning, 106
Lectins, 2
Left anterior descending coronary artery (LAD), 27
Left-sided heart failure, 30
Legionnaire's disease, 51
Leigh's syndrome, 68, 101
Leiomyoma, 83, 112
Lentigo maligna melanoma, 87
Lesch-Nyhan syndrome, 101
Leukemia, 17
Libman-Sacks endocarditis, 32
Linitis plastica, 42
Lipofuscin, 32
Lipoid nephrosis, 74
Lipomas, 110
Lipoxygenase pathway, 13
Liquefactive necrosis, 14
Liver, 37–38
Liver cirrhosis, 37–38
Lobar pneumonia, 51
Lobular carcinoma, 89
Lung abscess, 57
Lung tumors, 52–53, 112
Lutembacher's syndrome, 29
Lymphoblastic lymphoma, 17
Lymphocytes, 8

M

Macrocytic anemia, 5
Macrophages, 8
Malabsorption of upper GI, 45
Malignancy, 1–2
Malignant hypertension, 29
Malignant melanoma, 86–87, 111
Malignant mesothelioma, 54–55
Malignant transformations, 1
Mallory bodies, 40
Mallory-Weiss syndrome, 41, 101
Marasmus, 45
Marfan's syndrome, 101–102
Maturity onset diabetes mellitus, 66
MCH, 111
MCHC, 111
MCV, 111
Meconium ileus, 43
Medulloblastoma, 68
Megaloblastic anemia, 19, 42
Meig's syndrome, 81, 102
Melanoma, 86–87, 111
Melanin, 85
MEN type II, 59, 103
Meningioma, 67
Meningitis, 69
Mesothelioma, 54–55, 113
Metabolic acidosis, 23–24
Metabolic alkalosis, 24
Metastasis, 1
Metastatic calcification, 14
Microcytic anemia, 19
Minimal change disease, 74
Mole, 85
Mucopolysaccharidosis, 100, 101, 102
Multiple endocrine neoplasia syndrome (MEN type IIa), 59, 103
Multiple myeloma, 94, 112, 115
Multiple neurofibromatosis, 70
Multiple sclerosis (MS), 70
Muscular dysrophy, 94
Myelofibrosis, 91
Myeloperoxidase staining, 17
Myocardial infarct, 27
Myocardial infarction, 27
Myxedema, primary, 63
Myxoma, 29, 112

N

NADPH oxidase, 21
Napkin-ring constriction, 47
Native American Indian, 36
Necrotizing cervicitis, 81
Neimann-Pick disease, 107
Neonatal respiratory distress syndrome (NRDS), 56
Nephritic syndrome, 73
Nephritis, 74
Nephrosis, 74
Nephrotic syndrome, 74
Neurofibrillary tangles, 67
Neutrophils, 8
Newborn intestinal obstruction, 43
Niacin deficiency, 4
Night blindness, 3
Nipple eczematoid lesion, 88
Non-Hodgkin's lymphoma, 16–17
Null cells, 8

O

Oat cell carcinoma, 52–53
Oligodendroglioma, 67
Osteoarthritis, 93
Osteochondromas, 92
Osteomalacia, 95
Osteomyelitis, 95
Osteoporosis, 93
Osteosarcoma, 91–92, 112
Ovarian tumors, 80, 82
Ovaries, 80

P

Paget's disease, 89, 94
Pancoast syndrome, 56, 102
Pancreatic carcinoma, 35
Pancreatic ductal cells, 35
Pancreatic endocrine tumors, 35
Pancreatic insufficiency, 35
Pancreatitis, 35
Panhypopituitarism, 61
Panlobular emphysema, 52
Papillary thyroid cancer, 62–63, 112
Paradoxical embolism, 31
Parkinson's disease, 70–71
Parotid gland, 41, 112
Patau's syndrome, 102
Pellagra, 4
Pemphigus, 85
Peptic ulcer disease (PUD), 42
Peptic ulcers, 42
Pernicious anemia, 19, 42
Peutz-Jegher syndrome, 102
Phagocytic cells, 9
Pheochromocytoma, 50, 61
Phyllodes tumor, 88
Pigment stones, 36
Pilocytic astrocytoma, 67
Pituitary adenoma, 60
Pituitary glands, 59–62
Placenta previa, 84
Platelet aggregation, 12
Pleomorphic adenoma, 111
Pleuritis, 56
Plummer-Vinson syndrome, 41
Pneumococcal lobar pneumonia, 51
Pneumonia, 51
Poliomyelitis, 69
Polycystic renal disease, 78–79
Polycythemia vera, 12
Portal hypertension, 29
Postmortem clot, 33
Precancerous lesions, 106
Predictive value of positive lab test, 110
Presenile dementia, 68
Primary adrenal insufficiency, 59
Primary biliary cirrhosis, 36
Procallus, 95
Progressive systemic sclerosis, 22
Prolactinoma, 112
Prostatic specific antigen (PSA), 82
Prothrombin time (PT), 11
Prussian blue reaction, 20

Pseudomembranous colitis, 44
Pseudomembranous enterocolitis, 44
Pseudomonas aeruginosa, 33
Pseudomyxoma peritonei, 107
Psoriasis, 86
Pulmonary emphysema, 52
Pulmonary hypertension, 49
Pulmonary thromboembolism, 49
Purulent meningitis, 69
Pyridoxine, 3

R

Rabies, 109
Radiation sickness, 109
Radiation therapy, 88
Ranula, 41
Raynaud's disease, 22
Reiter's syndrome, 92, 102
Renal calculi, 78
Renal failure, 75–76, 114
Renal infarct, 77
Renal insufficiency, 75
Renal papillary necrosis, 76
Renal tubulointerstitial lesions, 76
Renin, 77
Respiratory acidosis, 24
Respiratory alkalosis, 25
Respiratory distress syndrome (RDS), 55–56
Reticulocytes, 14–15
Reye's syndrome, 102
Rh, 20
Rheumatic fever, 27–28
Rheumatic heart disease, 28
Rheumatoid arthritis, 96
Rickets, 3, 4, 95

S

Sanfilippo's syndrome, 102
Sarcoidosis, 54
Sarcomas, 2, 89–90

Schistosomiasis, 80
Secondary tuberculosis, 51
Sensitivity, 110
Sequestrum, 93
Sertoli-Leydig cell tumor, 80
Serum alkaline phosphatase, 92
Serum creatinine, 111
Serum hCG, 105
Sezary syndrome, 103
Sheehan's syndrome, 103
Shock, 32
Sickle cell anemia, 19
Sigmoid diverticula, 46
Silicosis, 54
Singer's nodules, 55
Sipple's syndrome, 59, 103
Sjogren's syndrome, 22, 103
Small cell carcinoma of the lung, 52–53
Small cell lung cancer, 52–53
Specificity, 110
Splenomegaly, 38, 40
Squamous cell carcinoma, 86, 111
Squamous cell carcinoma of lung, 53
Squamous papillomas, 54
Staghorn (struvite) calculi, 78
Staining, 109
Steatorrhea, 47
Stein-Levanthal syndrome, 82, 103
Subdural hematoma, 69, 106
Sudden infant death syndrome (SIDS), 103
Systemic lupus erythematosus (SLE), 22, 75

T

T3 resin uptake test, 64
T3 suppression test, 64
Tabes dorsalis, 67
Takayasu's arteritis, 31
Tay-Sachs disease, 106–107
Testicular tumors, 81
Tetralogy of Fallot, 30

Thiamine deficiency, 3, 5
Thrombocytopenia, 11
Thrombotic thrombocytopenic purpura (TTP), 11
Thymic neoplasms, 62
Thymoma, 62
Thyroid cancer, 62–63
Thyroid carcinoma, 63
Toxic megacolon, 44
Traction diverticulum, 42
Transitional cell carcinoma, 79, 80
Transmural bowel infarcts, 47
Transudates, 23
Tropical sprue, 45
Tuberculosis, 51
Tuberculous arthritis, 96
Tumor promoters, 1
Turner's syndrome, 103
Type I diabetics, 66
Type II diabetics, 66

U

Ulcerative colitis, 44
Uremia, 76
Urinary tract infections, 79
Uterine choriocarcinoma, 83

V

Vetricular septal defect (VSD), 30
Viral hepatitis, 38
Viral intestinal pneumonia, 51

Vitamin A deficiency, 3, 4
Vitamin C deficiency, 4, 6
Vitamin D, 3
Vitamin D deficiency, 3
Vitamin E, 3, 4
Vitamin K, 3, 10
Vitamin K deficiency, 3, 5
Volvulus, 47
von Recklinghausen's disease, 70
von Willebrand's disease, 11

W

Waldenstrom's macroglobulinemia, 95
Waterhouse-Friderichsen syndrome, 104
Wegener's granulomatosis, 50
Wernicke's encephalopathy, 69
Wernicke-Korsakoff syndrome, 5
Whipple's disease, 44
Wilm's tumor, 80, 112
Wilson's disease, 40
Wound healing, 6

X

X-linked inheritance, 109
Xeroderma pigmentosum, 87

Z

Zenker's diverticulum, 41
Zollinger-Ellison syndrome, 42

Notes

ISBN 0-07-038216-6

Color Plates

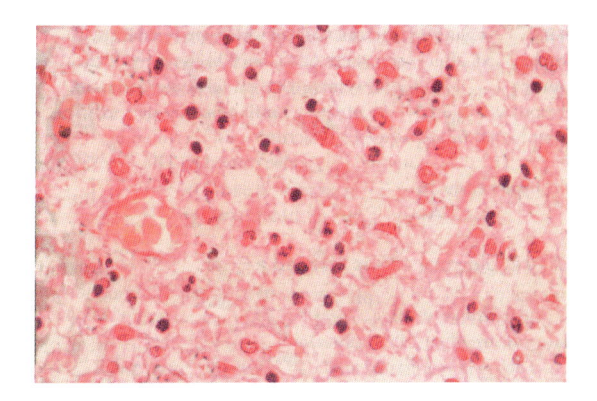

Color Plate 1 Inflammatory cells.

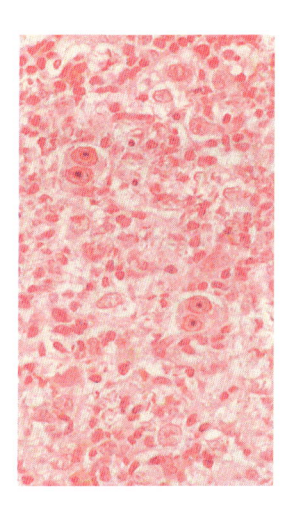

Color Plate 2 Reed Sternberg cells.

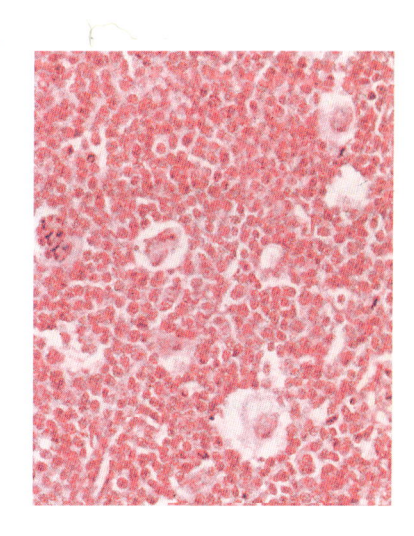

Color Plate 3 Burkitt's lymphoma.

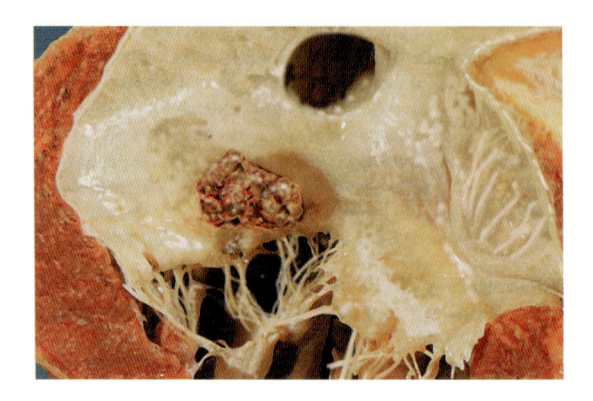

Color Plate 4 Heart valve thrombotic vegetations.

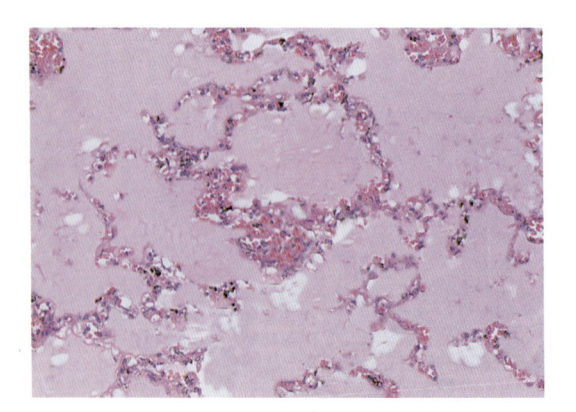

Color Plate 5 Pulmonary edema.

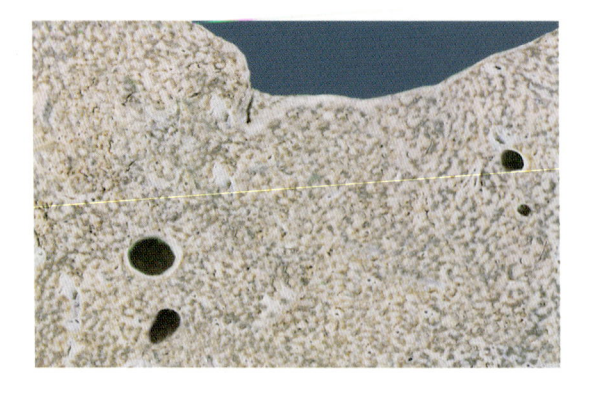

Color Plate 6 "Nutmeg liver" or congested liver.

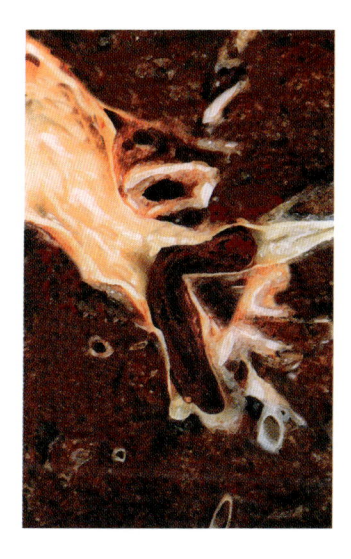

Color Plate 7 Embolism from lower leg to lung.

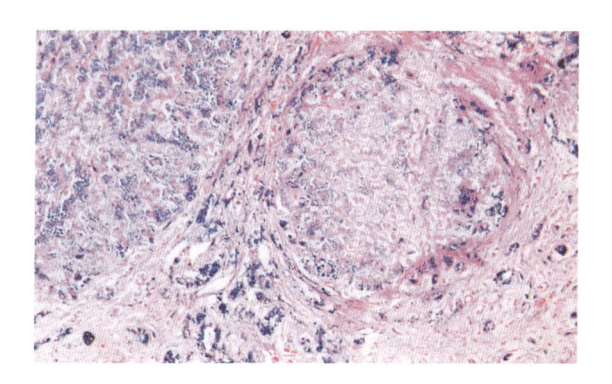

Color Plate 8 Hemochromatosis.

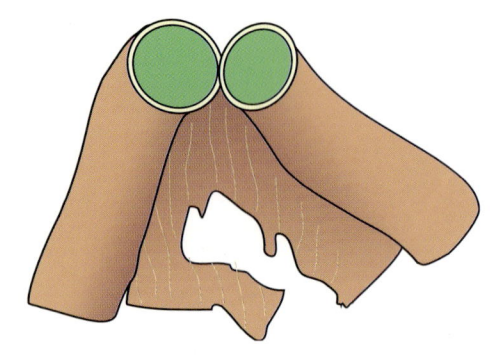

Color Plate 9 Meconium ileus.

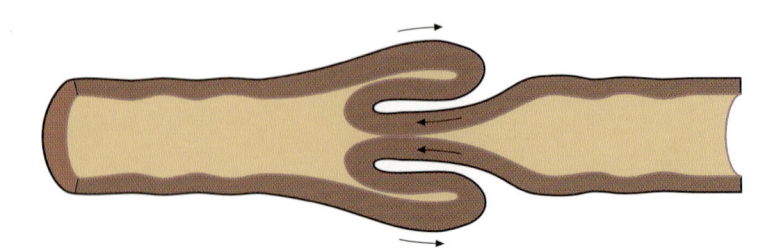

Color Plate 10 Intussusception.

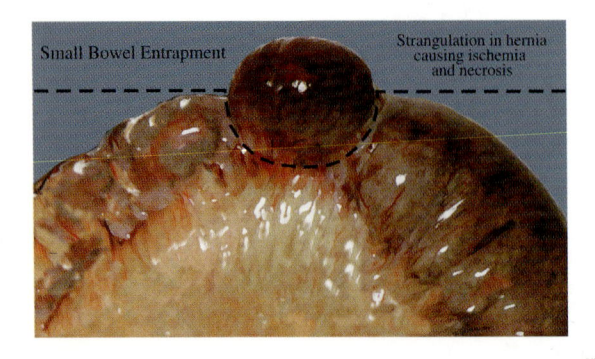

Color Plate 11 Necrosis of bowel by hernial strangulation.

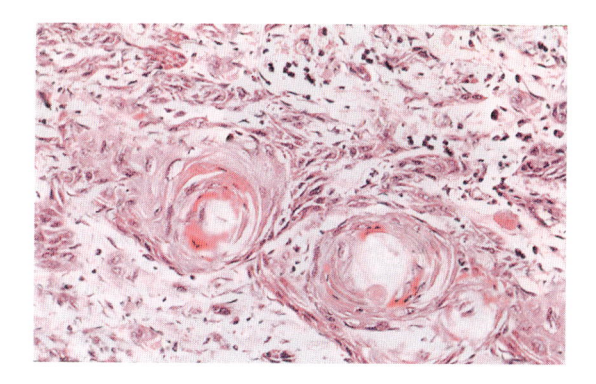

Color Plate 12 Squamous cell carcinoma of the lung.

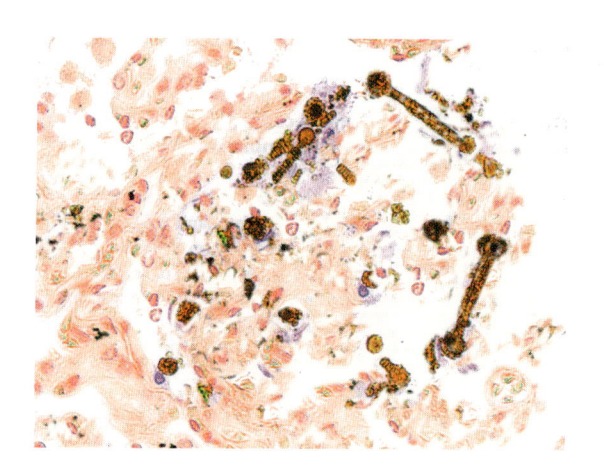

Color Plate 13 Asbestos bodies.

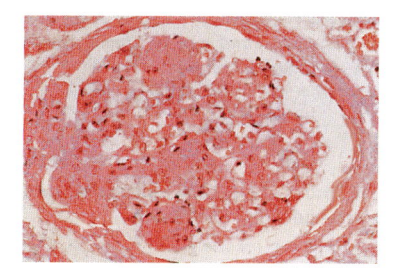

Color Plate 14 Nodular glomerulosclerosis.

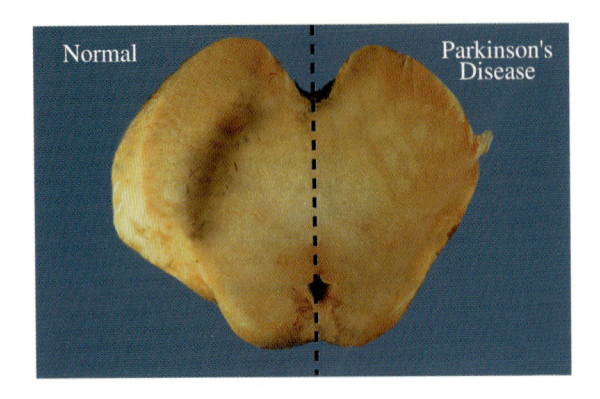

Color Plate 15 Normal versus Parkinson's disease.

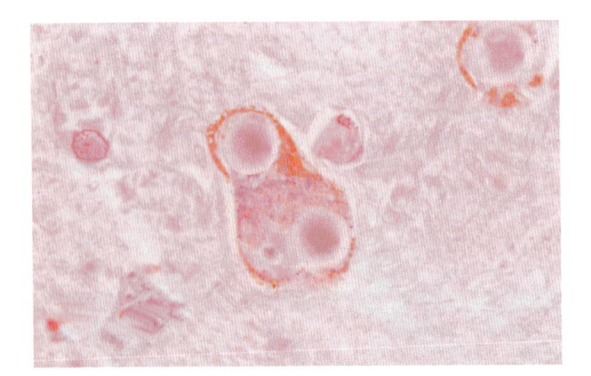

Color Plate 16 Lewy body found in Parkinson's disease.

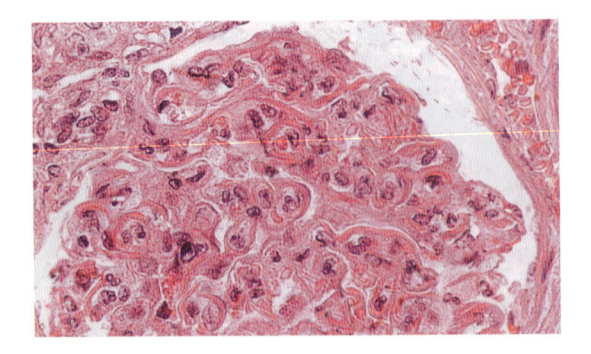

Color Plate 17 Lupus nephropathy.

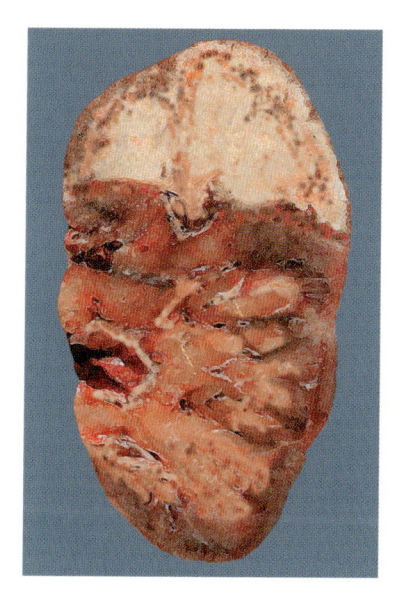

Color Plate 18 Renal infarct.

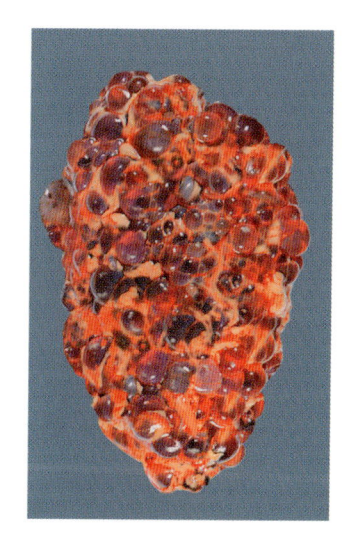

Color Plate 19 Adult polycystic disease of the kidney.

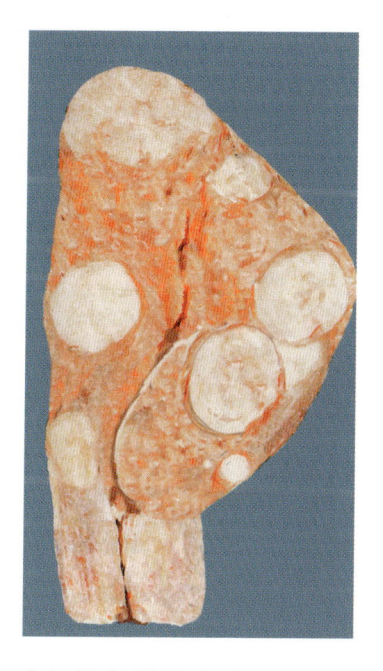

Color Plate 20 Uterine leiomyoma.

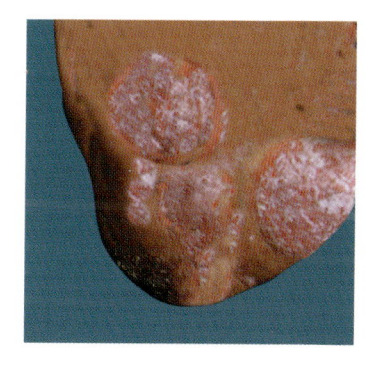

Color Plate 21 Psoriasis at elbow.

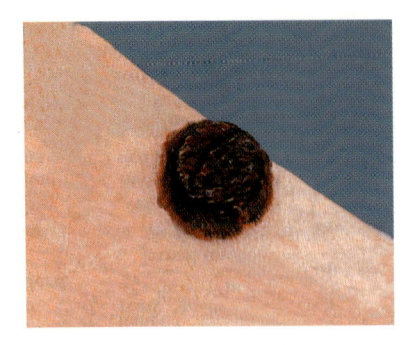

Color Plate 22 Malignant melanoma.

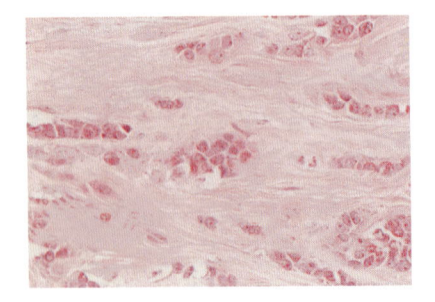

Color Plate 23 Invasive lobular breast cancer.

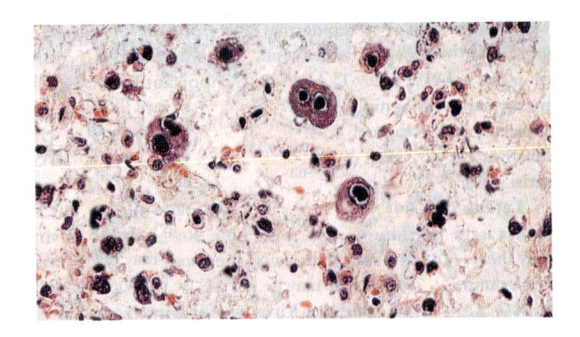

Color Plate 24 CMV inclusion bodies.